METABOLISM MADE SIMPLE

METABOLISM

MADE

SIMPLE

MAKING SENSE OF NUTRITION TO
TRANSFORM METABOLIC HEALTH

SAM MILLER

LIONCREST
PUBLISHING

METABOLISM MADE SIMPLE

Making Sense of Nutrition to Transform Metabolic Health

FIRST EDITION

ISBN   978-1-5445-3417-6 *Hardcover*
         978-1-5445-3418-3 *Paperback*
         978-1-5445-3419-0 *Ebook*

For my readers: Looking back on my health and fitness journey, I realize that these pursuits served as a gateway to immeasurable personal development and marked the start of discovering my own true potential as a human. While it may seem like fitness or fat-loss goals are "surface level" pursuits, I am confident that, when taken seriously, your health and fitness practices will plant the seeds for future personal growth and, in time, allow you to become the best version of yourself.

Thank you for allowing me to be a part of your journey to reach your goals, and thank you for reading this book.

CONTENTS

DISCLAIMER

This book is for entertainment and general informational purposes only and does not constitute the practice of medicine, nursing or other professional health care services, including the giving of medical advice, and no doctor–patient or coach–client relationship is formed.

The use of information on this book, related notes, and images and/or the reliance on the information provided is to be done at the user's own risk. The content of this book is not intended to be a substitute for professional medical advice, diagnosis, or treatment and is for educational purposes only.

Always consult your physician before beginning any exercise or nutrition program and users should not disregard, or delay in obtaining, medical advice for any medical condition they may have, and should seek the assistance of their health care professionals for any such conditions.

By accessing this book, the reader/listener acknowledges that the entire contents and design of this book are the property of

Oracle Athletic Science LLC, or used by Oracle Athletic Science LLC with permission, and are protected under US and international copyright and trademark laws.

Except as otherwise provided herein, users of this book may save and use information contained in the book only for personal or other non-commercial, educational purposes. No other use, including, without limitation, reproduction, retransmission or editing, of this book may be made without the prior written permission of Oracle Athletic Science LLC.

By accessing this book, the reader acknowledges that Oracle Athletic Science LLC makes no warranty, guarantee, or representation as to the accuracy or sufficiency of the information featured in this book and the reader understands that like any topic or genre information may change over time and it is the reader's responsibility to stay abreast of these changes as research and industry practices evolve.

Trademarks:

The acronym and term "SHREDS™" Biofeedback methodology is protected for Class 41 and Class 44 use by US and international trademark law.

INTRODUCTION

As early as my high school days, my favorite men's health magazines had me convinced that eating yogurt and walnuts every day at 10:00 a.m. was the secret sauce to achieving the body of my dreams. The ten-minute break between classes meant I had just enough time to rush to my locker for my fitness magazine-approved "healthy" snack. To be honest, I didn't even really like walnuts at the time.

Day in and day out, I thought this template was the recipe for success with my fitness goals. I assumed there was something magical about that specific combination of foods and eating them at that specific time. Surely if I deviated, I would instantly lose all my gains or add five pounds of pure fat.

No one taught me that someone else's ideal list of foods does not need to be the same as my ideal list of foods. Not all foods will be ones you enjoy or ones that make you feel good, and not all will fit your nutritional budget. Exhibit A: I now rarely eat walnuts, and this 10:00 a.m. snack time wouldn't work in my current life full of podcast recordings, public speaking, and

Zoom meetings. Not that there's anything wrong with walnuts, but this approach was restrictive and uninformed. These patterns of restriction resulted in lost muscle and energy as well as a lesser quality of life due to my lack of education around metabolism, calories, and macronutrients.

While I no longer eat yogurt and walnuts at 10:00 a.m., I see the same problems perpetuated in the health and fitness industry and in diet culture. We are inundated with overstated promises, "shortcuts," and "quick fix" propaganda. Not to mention every individual is subject to overhearing the watercooler talk at the office or seeing a friend's latest vegan recipe post on Pinterest. The clients I've served over the years may not come to me setting their watches to consume their snacks at 10:00 a.m., but they often find their way to my digital doorstep after counting points, eliminating carbs, eliminating animal foods, falling for fads, or following a rigid meal plan of some kind.

The truth is, "health foods" will always be relative to our goals, energy demands, digestive health, and mental state. All of these factors comprise the complex and seemingly amorphous concept of metabolism, which we will unpack together. There's no secret stuff. Some approaches may be slightly more optimal or advantageous than others, but your ability to adhere to a plan rooted in your personal preferences and some of the evidence-based strategies that I will outline will serve you better than program hopping to the latest fad diet flavor of the week.

I've spent the last fifteen-plus years identifying the most important factors when it comes to nutrition, transformation, and metabolic health for myself, my clients, and the coaches that I mentor so that you don't have to. Aside from my own health and transformation experiences mentioned above, I've coached countless individuals in their journey, as well as leading over 2,500 coaches in their efforts to help others through fitness and nutrition coaching. I started learning about personal training my senior year of high school and spent the decade that followed reading book after book, obtaining certification after certification, and coaching client after client. This process started just before my college years. During that time, I coached clients of all shapes, sizes, and fitness skillsets in person by working at a variety of gyms, campus recreation centers, and corporate wellness facilities. I even started coaching clients online during my master's degree as early as 2012 before it was "the cool thing to do" on Instagram. All of these influential experiences facilitated the development of the concepts that I will share with you in this book. I continue to work in the industry as a board-certified and credentialed health practitioner, where my focus and specialty is providing continuing education for health, fitness, and nutrition professionals through my programs. I also host one of the industry's top nutrition podcasts called *Sam Miller Science*, which you can find and download on Apple Podcasts, Spotify, and Amazon Music.

Unlike most authors in the diet, nutrition, or fitness industry, I am not writing this book to sell a diet or a specific exercise program. In this book, you won't find a seven-day fix or a gimmick that sounds too good to be true. In fact, we won't talk a ton about tactics or schemes. Instead, this book pulls back the curtain on why many diets fail and the science behind fixing the common pitfalls that exist for dieters, along with the tools I've used to educate fitness coaches and health professionals. This is not a "done for you" book. This is a guide to climb the proverbial mountain of your choice and to serve as your spotter to protect against preventable pitfalls in the diet industry. You will not be given a cookie-cutter meal plan or one-size-fits-all exercise routine. If that is why you picked up this book, I simply cannot oblige, as it would exacerbate the current state of the industry. The health, fitness, and nutrition industry is saturated with tactics and programs that fail to teach principles or the necessary critical thinking skills. Even the programs that are not ripe with misinformation often fail to build autonomy or allow for freedom of thought, or freedom of choice. The approaches and evidence in this book are based on over a decade of working with individuals from all walks of life and tailoring approaches that were best suited for their unique journey. This book also draws upon research and supporting evidence in the field. Last, but not least, you will also find notes on my fifteen-plus years of mistakes from my own health and fitness escapades.

My goal in the chapters that follow is to simplify the nuance and intricacies of metabolism while expanding your dietary horizons beyond what Slim Fast Sally, Weight-Watching Wilma, or Ketogenic Kevin have told you that you need to do to achieve dietary success.

When we zoom in on individual research, we see that any diet has the potential to work when we account for the primary transformation variables. Or more specifically, when we equate calories and protein, we see similar progress in the pursuit of fat loss. Research is fantastic, but even research studies can add to the confusion of diet-related noise, ultimately leading to us spinning our wheels once again. And if we are being honest, most of us are not picking up the latest scholarly journal publication or getting email updates on the most recent research from exercise physiology labs or getting the scoop on nutrition studies conducted in metabolic wards.

Most of the aforementioned dietary interventions work for a period of time, but there's a problem: they don't work forever. This might seem contradictory given the statements above, but it's what we have learned from weight loss research: there is limited evidence for long-term weight maintenance after a "successful" initial diet or weight-loss phase; in fact the majority of individuals regain more weight than they lose on their initial diet attempt. This is incredibly well exemplified by a study of participants from the NBC show *The Biggest Loser*. Participants not only struggled to maintain their weight, but many of them regained the *vast majority* of the weight they originally lost during their participation in the show.[1]

This might come as a surprise to you, but it is in alignment with other diet industry research. Other studies show that dieters regain 35% of weight lost in an intervention after one year, and they regain the majority of weight lost after five years.[2] Evidence for long-term maintenance is not absent from research or scientific literature, but it is relatively scarce. Two factors that should be considered in this discussion are how you define "successful weight loss" and what you might consider to be "long-term" weight loss. Both of these terms hinge upon the individual and our ability to align nutrition and dietary practices with their metabolic status quo. For example, losing ten pounds and keeping it off for ten months is different from losing one hundred pounds and keeping it off for ten years.

In this book, you will learn about metabolism and nutrition, but most importantly, you will learn how to determine the best approach depending on the variables that contribute to present metabolic status. You can even become nutritionally agnostic if you choose. If nothing else, we must stop adapting the person to the most popular diet approach at any given moment and start adapting proven dietary approaches and principles to the person. A successful nutritional intervention can promote metabolic health, extend lifespan, and provide newfound confidence. But execution is often difficult, and when we diet repeatedly in an improper fashion, not only do we often fail to make the progress we desire, but we risk losing some of these potential benefits—or, worse yet, doing harm to ourselves.

Most health, fitness, nutrition, and diet books have a plan, program, or membership to sell you upon completion. This book does not. Rather than commoditizing a particular strategy, my goal is that you can have freedom to participate in whatever eating style best matches your lifestyle, preferred activities, desired quality of life, and current internal health status. This may or may not be the approach that you are currently following.

The book will begin with a foray into diet culture and its common preventable pitfalls, followed by a ten-thousand-foot view of how your metabolism works and demystifying common myths. Once we have the blueprint for connecting the dots and making individualized dietary decisions, we will discuss some recipes for success when it comes to managing metabolism and maximizing health.

PART 1

UNDERSTANDING NUTRITION, DIET CULTURE, AND METABOLISM

DOING AWAY WITH DIET CULTURE

Over a period of three years from 2013 to 2016, the National Health and Nutrition Examination Survey reported 49.1% of adults in the US had tried to lose weight in the previous twelve months, including 56.4% of women and 41.7% of men. Among adults who had tried to lose weight, the most commonly reported methods were exercising (62.9%) and eating less food (62.9%), followed by consuming more fruits, vegetables, and salads (50.4%).[3]

The commoditization of diets and diet culture has only exacerbated these statistics and circumstances since 2016. We are marketed to and manipulated in such a way that we are sapped of attention and financial resources as we continue to buy into the latest fad or gimmick that promises to shed the pounds for good, all while lining the pockets of and feeding those who make false or overstated promises of fat-loss success. Unfortunately, most people who aspire to lose weight exist in what feels like Oz, with a man behind the curtain, or perhaps even the 1999 film *The Matrix*. Much like Morpheus presenting Neo with the opportunity to see the truth or remain the same, we must leave behind the overstated promises and false reality and embrace some cornerstone nutritional principles (our red pill solution to diet culture).

We are bombarded with inaccurate messaging around metabolism and fad approaches that simply do not work over a long trajectory. Antiquated "wisdom" around the idea of calories, energy, and traditional diets—and, more specifically, their execution—has failed our society. I call this linear subtraction of calories and increase in activity level "downhill dieting" because there's never a pause or an attempt to prevent the metabolic downregulation that occurs as we attempt to achieve fat loss. This method where calories are subtracted and activity is increased has failed our society, as evidenced by the dietary rebound statistics. It's not that we shouldn't diet, count calories, or exercise, but we need to understand how to leverage, manipulate, and time these tools properly to achieve long-term results.

Most people making any type of foray into the fitness space are seeking fat loss or muscle gain. For every handful of people seeking fat loss or aesthetic improvements, you might see one person who is dieting for other reasons—maybe to perform better at the gym or live longer or because they had a scary visit to the doctor's office.

Each year, we recycle approaches, and a brave bunch of New Year's resolutioners take a stab at a new diet, or they repeat the same diet that never worked before. We see repeated attempts with fad diets—Whole30, paleo, low-carb, low-fat, keto, etc. It only takes one trip to the grocery store or department store to see a smattering of magazines or catalogs of quick fixes.

Sally saw J-Lo on the *Today* show talking about eating zero carbs and her other favorite celebrity, Gwyneth Paltrow, talking about intuitive fasting, so she decides to combine the two. She thinks, *This is it! I am finally going to get the weight off for good!* She grabs the magazine, scribbles some notes, and approaches the week ahead with an extra bit of zeal toward her body goals so that she can finally drop those two dress sizes. After a week, Sally has lost a few pounds, but now she wonders what comes next. Does she diet forever?

The problem with many of the popular dietary approaches is they fail to take into account the metabolic consequence of prolonged dieting. What often happens is:

- Sally gets stuck eating a ridiculously low-calorie and low-nutrient diet because she thinks it's the only way to go, and she falls into a hole of metabolic adaptation and deficiency;
- Sally pushes down her cravings until they erupt mid-diet attempt, and she ends up emptying her cabinets in a whirlwind binge during a momentary lapse of willpower; and/or
- Sally ultimately goes back to the way she was eating because she doesn't have the tools to do otherwise, and the weight (which was mostly water weight anyway) comes right back.

Sometimes oversimplifying diets with general guidelines breeds widespread understanding. Other times oversimplification leaves portions of the population spinning their wheels en route to their goals. Food not only contains energy; food is analogous to having a pre-packaged set of instructions for your metabolism, each nutrient a tool to be used at the right time and place to drive a specific result. You could think of this as an individualized, demand-based approach to nutrition. For example, protein is not only great for satiety and managing appetite; it also promotes recovery and stimulates muscle protein synthesis (in other words, it builds muscle). Protein also has a relatively high thermic effect compared to other macronutrients, meaning the body burns more calories processing protein than other macronutrients (more on this later).

Calories in vs. calories out is a great starting point for the elementary elements of energy balance, especially for those who are overweight or obese with a history of overeating and underexercising. Calorie and macronutrient counting is a way to control the variable of energy intake on a daily basis, but this is a slippery slope.

The majority of the population in the United States and Western society, in general, tends to be overfed but undernourished, meaning that while we consume calorie-dense choices, those foods are not always dense in micronutrients, vitamins, and minerals, or they may not contain the proper amounts of essential fats and amino acids for optimal health. We will discuss the topic of calories and macronutrients in future sections, as well as other key nutritional definitions and principles.

In opposition to chronic dieters, we have a subset of society that trends toward overindulgence in hyperpalatable, high-calorie foods. While I'm holistically in favor of a little break to celebrate your four-year-old's birthday or occasionally enjoying your favorite treat, that isn't the problem here. The problem is the compounding interest of poor food choices on a meal-by-meal and day-to-day basis paired with inactivity. This results in the issues associated with the hypercaloric standard American diet (SAD), including metabolic syndrome and insulin resistance, along with a plethora of other conditions.

The primary issue with a static glance at energy intake and energy expenditure is that your metabolism is not a static being. It is in constant survey mode, observing the energy we expend, the energy we take in via our diet, and the energy we have stored as body fat. It is an energy regulator, and it excels at its job, whether we underfeed or overfeed relative to our baseline needs.

Hard-wired into our physiology, we have the ability to assess multiple forms of stress or energy threats, such as stress from a job, circadian stress from lack of sleep or adequate sun exposure, or internal stress like inflammation. The body then adapts and compensates accordingly. This is where terms like *metabolic adaptation* and *metabolic compensation* stem from. Not only will the body compensate with changes in hunger, cravings, and other sensations, but it will slow metabolic rate down. Again, this metabolic decline varies from person to person, but it does happen in response to stress and energy threats like chronic dieting in modern society.

Generally speaking, most dieters add more stress (more exercise and less food) without any type of seasonality or planned adjustments in their approach. Metabolism, as a miser of calories, can become more efficient or inefficient to meet the demands imposed upon it simply to keep us alive (more on this in our adaptive physiology section). Without metabolism's adaptability, our species would have been extinct many food shortages ago. Conversely, with less exercise and more eating, we also place the body under stress, which results in us developing excessive amounts of fat tissue, insulin resistance, and metabolic syndrome. In many cases, we've lost sight of "nutrition" in a world of fad diets and super-sized fries.

Over time, we develop a metabolic identity that is a predictor of our future success or failure with any dietary approach or protocol. We each have a metabolic fingerprint characterized by our past choices. Tom, who really likes Twinkies and hasn't touched a dumbbell since his teens, has a vastly different state of internal health than Tanya, who likes tempeh, tai-chi, and total body workouts.

While these two avatars may seem like two entirely different species because of their habits, humans all have similar governing rules and adaptive physiology by which our bodies operate. However, as we age, each decision that we make and each day that passes contributes to the development of this metabolic fingerprint or identity. Think of how the act of water repeatedly passing through dirt or sand forms its shape over time. This concept is paramount because understanding metabolic uniqueness overrides any fad diet, advice, or coaching protocol you find on the internet.

In sum, your body and your metabolism are products of past and present physiology, as well as your perceptions around food and exercise. We all have unique identities. One of my colleagues, Dr. Jade Teta, explains that "just as each human varies in their physical appearance, we vary in our metabolic function as well." Of course, this is not to say that appearance is the driver of metabolism. In fact, you would likely argue the opposite.

You see, it isn't just about your current diet. It is about creating awareness from your past decisions and leveraging that awareness to create present and future success with a diet of your choice. If we look at the diet industry as a whole, there are a host of problems that can be solved with a few evidence-backed solutions:

Problem: Most nutrition or "health-related" advertising or propaganda is packaged as a diet, and the non-diet nutrition world is filled with hyperpalatable, calorie-dense foods that lack micronutrients.

Solution: Understand that even at the grocery store, you are being marketed to, and products are positioned for sell-through purposes, not health purposes.

Problem: The media and most dietary approaches fail to educate people about metabolism.

Solution: Understand that a diet is simply a collective set of practices or an approach that manipulates your nutrition in an attempt to create desired results.

Problem: The adaptability of nutrition gets lost, and we are stuck with specific dietary approaches or eating structures based on what has been marketed to us.

Solution: Understand that nutrition can be used and manipulated to achieve any goal, which means you can create the best diet for you instead of relying on a specific diet's overstated promises.

Problem: For some it is eating based on rules defined by colored Tupperware, for others it is a framework of food choices characterized by eating butter with your bacon, but in either case the problem is many individuals take action without understanding basic tools of the nutritional trade like macronutrients and micronutrients.

Solution: Learn about the seasonality of dieting, or periodization, which means we can manipulate nutrition to achieve any goal.

Beyond these problems, there's arguably more false information in the fitness industry than any other. From somewhat well-intended but biased philosophies lacking evidence (such as eating more frequent meals to "stoke the metabolic fire") to straight fabrication of facts (like needing a magical metabolism "reset"), the industry always has a trendy solution for all of our fitness woes.

The only way to break free from these tempting instant-gratification traps is to truly understand metabolism and its most integral components. Your metabolism is adaptable and can change based on what you eat and your activity level. Your metabolism is not broken. This is not a surgical wound or battle scar, but it will take science, skill, strategy, and some effort to improve over time.

In the chapters that follow, we will begin to make sense of metabolism and explore why current approaches to dieting and industry terminology may be misaligned with your metabolic makeup, leading to confusion and uncertainty.

WHAT IS METABOLISM ANYWAY?

Let's start with the basics: you eat food to nourish your cells. If you make poor food choices, you may compromise not only your physical appearance, but the health of your cells and your quality of life. Metabolism is the chemical processes that occur within a living organism in order to maintain life. However, if you asked most people about their metabolism, the answers would look quite different.

In over a decade of coaching clients en route to their transformation goals, I've found that most people tend to define metabolism only in terms of speed. You can probably remember a childhood friend from grade school who was thin as a rail and seemingly ate whatever they wanted—and this individual was labeled as having a fast metabolism. You may have also had a friend who was overweight or carried a little bit more fat than the average child and was deemed to have a slow metabolism, but there is more to the story than these labels.

As we learned in the last chapter, our metabolism is adaptive. This means that as a system, it considers environmental stressors, energy availability, and output on an indefinite basis to ensure our survival. Scientists as early as Darwin observed that natural history is shaped by the struggle for resources. Because there was never enough food to go around, species evolved under conditions of scarcity. With too much stress, too much food, or too little food, our body will create survival-driven adaptations—some more desirable than others. This is known as *adaptive physiology*. Remember: we're extremely complex living organisms in an equally complex, ever-changing environment. In the subsequent sections, we will discuss why our metabolism, much like our ancestors' metabolisms, is adaptive and how to manage it to achieve our health, fitness, or fat-loss goals.

MAKING SENSE OF METABOLISM

Does adaptive physiology still apply to a human being in 2021 and beyond? Yes.

While your body is advanced, miraculous, and complex in its own way, it does not precisely "understand" fitness or fad diets. For example, it doesn't see CrossFit or the ketogenic diet. To make sense of CrossFit or keto, your body simply translates them as stimuli, energy availability, tension, load, stress, and relative nourishment. Remember this going forward because it will be a key component of understanding the various mechanisms by which the body reduces, manages, or regulates total hormonal or metabolic output.

Metabolism is a measure of the body's energy use but can also be used to describe the bodily system that operates and adjusts dynamically to maintain life. The system itself starts in your brain, sensing food, sun, heat, and activity, and it interacts with everything from your gut to receptors in all of your cells. Hormones are potent messengers related to metabolism as well (more on these later). These messages influence cellular behavior and the expression of certain genes. Your brain has a direct line to communicate with these different cells, glands, and organs to maintain bodily functions and survival. Your body has a massive blueprint: your complete genetic code. However, not all of this code is active and being built from at all times. Your internal and external environment decides what portion of the code gets turned on and what gets turned off. Your hormones are a part of this internal signaling and messaging; that is, they can directly influence what genes are turned on or expressed.

The key takeaway here is that metabolism is both an energy network and a feedback network, so it *does* perceive or "count calories," along with a multitude of other external signals, while continuously monitoring internal signals as well.

So, who or what senses these signals anyway? The answer lies in our neuroendocrine system: the interaction of the brain, pituitary, adrenals, and reproductive glands and tissues. All of these systems are stringently controlled by feedback mechanisms and pathways that communicate between the nervous system and the endocrine system. In many ways, these glands, tissues, cells, and signals create a biochemical supercomputer.

The way these communication pathways work is similar to how a thermostat controls the temperature in your home or vehicle. If the temperature is too warm, the thermostat detects this and turns on the air conditioning. Once the room cools down and the optimum temperature is reached, the thermostat turns off the air conditioning to prevent the temperature from dropping too low. This negative feedback mechanism keeps the temperature regulated in the house or vehicle. Similarly, negative feedback mechanisms within the neuroendocrine network prevent overactivity. When predetermined levels of these hormones are reached, the brain stops releasing hormones, thereby turning off the domino effect or trigger of hormone release.

Bear in mind, these hormones influence all of the primary systems involved in human physiology (including the cardiovascular, musculoskeletal, nervous, and immune systems). What makes the metabolism more complex is that it is constantly scanning and observing our external environment for stressors, while simultaneously evaluating our internal hormone levels using a system of checks and balances. While this scanning of external stressors or threats sounds archaic, remember we are hard-wired in the same manner as our ancestors. You'd probably want your body to be able to respond accordingly if you happened to turn a corner and spot a dangerous predator. Our physiology has changed minimally, but our societal demands, training stimuli, and nutritional strategies have changed at warp speed. Not to mention, most of us are a far cry from hunting and gathering our own beef or blueberries in nature.

Hundreds of thousands of years ago, the endocrine system had a very basic duty when it came to hormone production. Our ancestors' bodies needed adequate amounts of food, water, sleep, and sunlight to optimize hormonal function in order to survive. The human body knows better than to reproduce during times of extreme famine or stress or when facing scarcity of key resources. It makes hormonal and metabolic adaptations to hedge against these threats.

Any extremes serve as signals to adjust or halt hormonal production to conserve energy. For example, sex and reproduction require energy (something we want to conserve during times of scarcity). In a stressful or scarce environment, the chances of successfully breeding, carrying a child to term, and being able to feed an infant would be slim.

By downregulating hormone production, in a traditional, somewhat antiquated paleolithic sense, a man conserves energy for essential tasks like finding food and surviving. By having an absent menstrual cycle, a woman avoids the complications of having to devote massive amounts of energy to sustaining a growing fetus and breastfeeding a newborn child. This is very calorically costly, meaning it takes a lot of food to grow and feed a baby. Aside from reproductive hormones, downregulation in thyroid hormone helps prevent starvation by thwarting additional energy burn and ensuring resource preservation. The two most pivotal variables described in the aforementioned scenario are stress and energy. Our body must manage both interdependent variables not only to survive but to achieve dietary success. In Chapter 3, we will explore and define energy in nutritional terms including calories, macronutrients, and more so that we can better account for their influence on metabolic health and the transformation process.

ENERGY

One thing that all the world's botanical and animal life forms have in common is that we require energy to live. Human beings require energy for executive functioning, musculoskeletal movement, and basic survival requirements, like keeping blood circulating and generating body heat. While plants can use light to create energy through a process called photosynthesis, humans need to consume energy from food sources that contain calories and essential nutrients.

For those less familiar with our botanical friends, plants trap light energy with their leaves. Plants use the energy of the sun to change water and carbon dioxide into a sugar called glucose, which they use for energy and to make other substances like cellulose and starch. Animals also can use glucose as the body's fuel, but we are unable to create energy through photosynthesis. The digestible carbohydrates in our diet are converted into glucose molecules and then into energy through a series of chemical reactions. Adenosine triphosphate (ATP) is the primary energy currency in cells.

While there's no quiz on energy or ATP at the end of this chapter and we won't be entering a time warp to visit your high school biology professor, it is essential to understand the relationship between metabolism and energy. Consider energy in a few buckets. Humans have energy available to us via our daily diets as well as stored energy in our fat or muscle. The combination of these three contribute to what we'll refer to as energy availability for the human body. We also expend energy through living, breathing, and completing fundamental tasks. This contributes to our resting metabolic rate, a key component of total daily energy expenditure, or the amount of energy we use (or calories we burn) simply being alive.

Before we dive into the nitty gritty of energy availability and energy expenditure, it is important to understand how we measure energy. ATP is derived from calories. Similar to financial currency or the metric system, we use calories as a unit of measurement to describe or standardize amounts of food energy. While there are certainly a myriad of diet methods to choose from, most aim to create a deficit or reduction of calories by reducing certain food types or amounts.

The calorie was originally used as a measurement tool in physics and engineering and its origins had nothing to do with nutritional science. German scientist Julius Mayer and French scientists Nicholas Clement, P. A. Favre, and J. T. Silbermann referenced the calorie as much as thirty to fifty years before the thermodynamic calorie carryover to nutritional science in 1887, largely attributed to a chemist named Wilbur Atwater.

These gentlemen were not the impetus for the calorie-counting obsession that we have today, but their scientific discoveries served as the basis for people like Lulu Hunt Peters, who published a bestseller called *Diet and Health: With Key to the Calories* in 1918. For the first time in a popular text, she instructed people to start thinking about food in terms of calories. She asserted, "Hereafter, you are going to eat calories of food. Instead of saying, 'one slice of bread,' or 'a piece of pie,' you will say, '100 calories of bread,' or '350 calories of pie.'"[4]

Food calorie counts are derived from measurements calculated in a device called a bomb calorimeter. This device essentially burns the food in one chamber and calculates the calories from the temperature rise in a chamber of water surrounding the food chamber. The human body doesn't operate exactly like a bomb calorimeter. A simple calorie count doesn't encompass all the signals and information a specific food sends to the body or the micronutrients a food provides, but we can use this metric to help control our portions of food and to have a better understanding of the total energy we consume from the foods we eat on a weekly basis.

CALORIES AND NUTRIENTS

Other scientists and nutrition researchers have elaborated and expanded upon this to describe finer details of nutrition like macronutrients and micronutrients. Macronutrients are protein, fat, carbohydrate, and arguably alcohol. Micronutrients are nutrients needed in small amounts, such as vitamins and minerals that are essential for health and daily bodily processes.

From an energetic standpoint:

- Fat: 9 calories

- Carbohydrate: 4 calories
- Protein: 4 calories
- Alcohol: 7 calories

Beyond providing energy, each nutrient has its own unique contributing role when it comes to bodily functions.

FAT AND ESSENTIAL FATTY ACIDS

Our body requires essential fatty acids (EFAs) that not only provide energy but thwart disease. Many studies have positively correlated essential fatty acids with reduction of cardiovascular morbidity and mortality, optimal brain and vision functioning, and prevention of cancer, arthritis, hypertension, diabetes mellitus, and neurological/neuropsychiatric disorders. The benefits of essential fatty acids are not limited to adults. We also see essential fatty acids contribute to improved infant development. Beneficial health effects of EFAs may be mediated through several different mechanisms, including alteration in cell membrane composition and even gene expression.[5]

There are many different types of fatty acids that our bodies can create, but essential fatty acids must be obtained from diet. There are only two completely essential fatty acids; linoleic acid (an omega-6) and alpha-linoleic acid (an omega-3). There are "conditionally" essential fatty acids as well: eicosapentaenoic acid (EPA) and docosahexaenoic acid (DHA). These are omega-3 fatty acids that are critical for health. While alpha-linoleic acid can be converted to EPA and DHA in the body, this process is very inefficient in the vast majority of individuals, which is why it becomes a worthwhile consideration to obtain them from the diet.[6] When looking at omega-6 and omega-3 fatty acid intake, it is important to understand that there appears to be a relationship between an increased omega-6:omega-3 ratio and metabolic diseases. Anthropological data indicates that the ancestral diet was roughly 1:1 or 2:1 in terms of omega-6:omega-3 ratio, and this is believed to be ideal. Between 1935 and 1939, the omega-6:omega-3 ratio was 8.4:1. In 1985, this ratio was at least 10.3:1 and even as high as 12.4:1 in other calculations. Later, between 2001 and 2011, the average ratio of omega-6 to omega-3 was reported as between 15:1 and 17:1. Today, in Western diet styles, the estimated average ratio is as high as 22:1, which has correlated well with the same rise in obesity, cardiovascular disease, and autoimmune disease.[7]

Not only is it important to meet essential fatty acid minimum requirements, but it is also important to make sure you have enough fat in general for hormone health; low-fat diets (10–20% of calories from fat) have been associated with decreased testosterone in men and women and decreased estradiol in women.[8] Given that fats provide nine calories per gram, a low-fat diet can also contribute to relative energy deficiency if overall nutrient intake is not closely monitored.

PROTEIN

Another macronutrient of concern is protein. Protein triggers muscle protein synthesis and provides a higher level of satiety, limits weight regain, and helps with improvements in body composition and metabolic profile.

But what is protein, exactly? "Any of a class of nitrogenous organic compounds that consist of large molecules composed of one or more long chains of amino acids and are an essential part of all living organisms, especially as structural components of body tissues such as muscle, hair, collagen, etc., and as enzymes and antibodies."[9] For those of you who aren't lab rats or spending your day memorizing Merriam-Webster's dictionary or nutrition textbooks, protein is provided by foods such as meat, poultry, legumes, dairy, eggs, and some plants. It is an essential nutrient, which means we cannot survive for extended periods of time without consuming it. Protein contains essential amino acids, which are like building blocks for each protein molecule. There are twenty-one amino acids in total, but only nine are essential, meaning the body cannot synthesize them and they must be derived from food. An essential amino acid (EAA) deficiency causes a reduced rate of protein synthesis in cells and tissues, particularly skeletal muscle. We need a variety of proteins to:

- Digest and absorb dietary nutrients via the small intestine.
- Transport nutrients (including long-chain fatty acids, vitamin A, and iron) and other molecules like cholesterol and triglycerides in blood.
- Oxidize nutrients (including fatty acids and glucose) to water and carbon dioxide.

Consequently, deficiencies of EAAs and micronutrients (including vitamin A, iron, zinc, and folate) remain a major nutritional problem in poor regions of the world, where people are less likely to have access to adequate amounts of protein.[10]

To further emphasize the foundational importance of protein, not only does it offer a host of positive contributions metabolically, but it is quite difficult to gain body fat from the overconsumption of protein. In an eight-week study, resistance-trained men were instructed to consume 4.4g/kg protein per day in addition to their normal dietary habits, causing them to eat an 800-calorie surplus purely from protein. At the end of the study, they showed no significant changes in body weight, fat mass, fat free mass (fat free mass includes organs, water, and connective tissue), or percent body fat, which suggests it is likely very hard to put on fat mass solely from overeating protein.[11]

We also observed this in a tightly controlled study in 2012, in which twenty-five healthy volunteers ate a weight-stable diet for a time period within a metabolic ward (thirteen to twenty-five days) and then were overfed 40% extra calories (954 calories per day average). In this study, the surplus did not solely come from protein. There were three groups: 5% protein, 15% protein, and 25% protein. All groups gained similar amounts of fat mass; however, the 15% and 25% protein groups gained 2.87kg and 3.18kg of lean body mass (LBM), respectively, while the low-protein group did not gain any extra LBM. Energy expenditure increased 160 calories per day in the 15% protein group and 227 calories per day in the 25% protein group, while the low-protein group didn't increase energy expenditure.[12]

Now that we've gone over the myriad benefits of having high protein intake, many of you might be skeptical and wondering about your kidneys. Since the 1980s, the myth that high protein consumption causes kidney damage has been perpetuated (largely amongst Gen X'ers and baby boomers) without sufficient evidence to back it up. When you actually look at the data, you see the opposite. One 2018 study featured protein intakes as high as 3.3g/kg (nearly 1.5g/lb) over up to a year in some cases without indication of negative repercussions for kidney health. To put this in perspective, that would be similar to a 150-pound individual eating 225 grams of protein or a 225-pound individual eating over 330 grams of protein.[13]

Protein is a cornerstone nutrient in effective dietary approaches. Anyone who tells you otherwise is out of touch with the research and the real-world application of nutrition.

CARBOHYDRATE

The word *carbohydrate* is a trigger for some and a love-hate relationship for others. This is largely because carbohydrate is the only macronutrient with no established minimum requirement. Although many indigenous populations have thrived with carbohydrate as their main source of energy, others have done so with few (if any) carbohydrate-containing foods throughout much of the year (for example, traditional diets of the Inuit, Laplanders, and some Native Americans).

The large brain of modern humans is energetically expensive and requires a lot of calories to function, meaning it needs a disproportionate share of dietary energy compared with the brains of other mammals (even primates).

The first hunting and gathering societies were characterized by greater consumption of not only animal foods but other foods with greater carbohydrate availability than leaves—including ripe fruit, honey, and eventually cooked starchy foods such as potatoes, rice, and grains.[14] The higher nutrient and energy density of this diet allowed for evolution of a smaller gastrointestinal tract, offsetting the energy demands of the brain.[15]

In addition to providing a dense source of energy, carbohydrates also provide dietary fiber, which can be a tool in the arsenal of any dieter looking to manage hunger, energy levels, and cravings (more on this later). So, while some may argue that carbohydrates are not "essential," they do serve a role in the human diet, especially for active individuals because carbs provide fuel not only for the brain, but for working muscle as well.

Many exercise programs like CrossFit or strength training in general have a strong glycolytic component, meaning athletes and lifestyle enthusiasts use a carbohydrate- or glucose-based energy system to fuel these activities. Your body demands energy at different rates for different activities. When you're walking, your body demands energy at a very low rate. Increasing to a slow jog burns through energy slightly faster. Burst into an all-out sprint, and your body demands energy at an extremely high rate.

Energy can be made from fat, but it's a slower process and hits its bottleneck of energy production right around a moderately paced jog for most individuals. Once you pass this threshold, the body goes to a process called glycolysis, which provides fast energy but also requires glucose (carbohydrate). Talk to anyone who has been keto and doing CrossFit for a longer period of time; performance and well-being certainly suffer with low carbohydrate consumption and glycolytic exercise.

In addition to the performance benefits, carbohydrates also play a large role for the chronic dieter and stressed undereater who is heavily into the stages of metabolic adaptation. This is due in large part to the fact that carbohydrates help us mitigate the unwanted effects of the hormone cortisol, which can become rampant in high-stress activities or competition, as well as in highly stressed individuals. Carbohydrates can also help us increase leptin, a powerful hormone that we'll discuss in the "managing metabolic adaptation" section of this book.

While protein, fat, and carbohydrate all provide calories, they are all uniquely valuable to the human diet in different ways. We need to move beyond the calorie count to fully embrace and understand the context and nuance of nutrition and use these macronutrient groups to derive essential amino acids, omega-3 fatty acids, and dietary fiber. We'll talk more about the context of calories and look at energy more specifically in the sections that follow.

MORE THAN A
CALORIE COUNT

From the origin of the calorie to Atwater's application to nutrition science to modern proposed solutions of points, portions, or particular eating styles, what seems to get lost in our immersive calorie-counting diets is that calories require context. In life, we rarely make decisions about units of measurement without context. For example, the temperature might be above freezing, but we still want to know if it's raining or not. If we need to travel one hundred miles, we might want to be aware of things like available roads, public transit systems, topography, and weather. Strolling a mile on a sunny day in Kansas is different from a mile uphill in the snow in Colorado or a mile during hurricane season in Florida. Our nutritional choices are not exempt from this.

Hundreds of millions of people have tried to use calorie management to achieve weight loss, and according to a meta-analysis conducted by researchers at UCLA, only a minuscule percentage of those using a conventional calorie-restricted diet lose weight and keep it off. I refer to this discrepancy as the *fat-loss fallacy,* a misunderstanding of the body's response to changes in energy availability and energy expenditure.

In the United States and in countries across the world following Western diets, hundreds of millions of people are overweight or obese. Every year, millions of people attempt a calorie-restricted program to try to lose weight. Unfortunately, these eager individuals are often met with nothing more than myths and misinformation that cause frustration and endless wheel spinning. In addition, only a tiny portion of these people are able to lose weight and keep it off. The flaw is not so much the concept of energy balance or a calorie deficit but the strategies to successfully lose weight.

Before we concern ourselves with deploying specific strategies, we first must have a better conceptual understanding of metabolism, energy intake (nutrition), and energy expenditure (from basal metabolism and movement). To progress with clarity toward any health, fitness, or nutrition goal, we have to understand that food is energy, but our body also stores and utilizes energy.

First, we will dive into the idea of energy availability and its importance for both chronic dieters and those with more weight to lose and less dieting experience.

ENERGY AVAILABILITY

Energy is more readily accessible than ever before. Not only do we have high-calorie, hyperpalatable food choices at the ready and fast food chains on nearly every corner, but now Amazon and many other companies will deliver your groceries, just in case you don't have the gumption to leave the house. Couple this with Instacart, Uber Eats, Postmates, Grubhub, and OrderUp, and most Americans can have any savory or sweet treat in their hands in a matter of minutes, or hours at the most.

Despite these technical advances, it is critical to understand and remember points from previous chapters. We are operating with physiological technology comparable to a typewriter (or older) in an age of Apple products and novel software. This isn't to say the body isn't advanced. It is still incredibly complex, and even after years of studying health, fitness, nutrition, and physiology, I'm continuously amazed at its capabilities.

As we begin to discuss energy, we should first acknowledge the divergent scenarios that create differences in metabolic makeup. On one hand, we have individuals struggling with excess body weight, metabolic syndrome, and insulin resistance (type 2 diabetes). On the other hand, there seem to be more chronic dieters than ever before. This group has fallen into a pattern of chronic restriction and deprivation, along with attempting the latest fads to reach their fat-loss goals.

While these two scenarios are distinct cases with unique outcomes, both serve as examples to showcase stress imposed on the body via dietary options and energy availability. Both supplying the body with excess energy and depriving the body with inadequate energy for long periods of time are problematic. When it comes to quality of life and sustainable body composition, we must achieve the Goldilocks amount of energy availability and energy expenditure at different times or "seasons" (more on this concept later), depending on our goals and health status.

When a body is overfed for prolonged periods, perceived energy availability is high. The body's intake of energy, specifically excess consumption of calories from food, exceeds our ability to burn or store that energy. We hit a threshold in our ability to pull that energy through the system—like overfilling your gas tank, but with more dire consequences than getting fuel on the exterior paint. Overfeeding contributes to insulin resistance and metabolic syndrome, and if this state persists, our cells become "resistant" to this influx of energy, and the body develops representative disease states. Insulin resistance from continued overfeeding and sedentary lifestyles contributes not only to diabetes but also to hyperlipidemia, inflammation, elevated uric acid, polycystic ovarian disease, and cancer.

Chronic calorie restriction presents a different set of problems, largely due to low energy availability. Despite what you might think, the body is aware of what you're up to and can be quite thrifty with its energy utilization when it senses a lack of resources available. In the case of energy deprivation, when the body goes through prolonged periods of calorie restriction, we see problematic hormonal adaptations, including but not limited to the thyroid, reproductive hormones, and adrenal hormones. While dieting may seem less "life-threatening" than chronic overconsumption of food in terms of disease risk, it can have a detrimental impact on quality of life for both men and women. It also can significantly impact fertility, especially in cases of hypothalamic amenorrhea or anovulation, where women are not able to ovulate or in some cases achieve a healthy menstrual cycle at all. In terms of energy expenditure, the transient hormonal changes are often referred to as *adaptive thermogenesis* or metabolic adaptation. But for the chronic dieter, it feels a lot like dysfunction and frustration.

Each of the above cases is unique and requires a different nutritional strategy to restore optimal health and achieve any desired physical goals or aesthetic outcomes. In addition to understanding your body's perceived energy availability, creating the best protocol for your current state of metabolic health requires learning about energy expenditure, also referred to as the highly sought after "calorie burn."

ENERGY EXPENDITURE

For fat loss, it has been beaten into our heads that calories matter. Calories in vs. calories out is a great starting point for the elementary elements of energy balance, and for most people, following this practice means observing food consumption vs. exercise activity or the simple breakdown of food consumption vs. movement. This leads to many individuals trying to exercise their way to lean, healthy bodies. We have found ourselves in a situation where gym memberships are at all-time highs, and there are more boutique fitness options and studios than ever before. Whether you fancy yourself some Orangetheory, F45, Soul Cycle, Flywheel, or the latest flavor of fitness that will be invented long after the creation of this book, you have no shortage of options available when it comes to getting your sweat on and burning some calories.

This begs the question: with all of these workout options at our disposal, why are we not leaner, fitter, and in better metabolic condition than ever before? One theory behind obesity is that we simply move less than our ancestors and that if we just exercise more, move more, and get more active, we will achieve long-term weight-loss success. After all, regular exercise has a ton of well-documented benefits, from cardiovascular health to immune and brain function. It also helps suppress chronic inflammation, which has been linked to both cardiovascular disease and autoimmune disorders.

However, exercise alone has not proven to be an effective tool when it comes to losing weight and keeping it off. Where exercise seems to shine is for weight maintenance or sustaining your physique *after* an initial period of weight loss. The exercise-only approach often fails because we can easily overconsume and out-eat our exercise efforts, and for some, large volumes of exercise trigger even more intense appetite sensations. Attempting to out-exercise our calorie consumption neglects key insights and discoveries from evolutionary anthropologists pertaining to metabolism and the constraints in calorie burn.

One large barrier to assessing the theory of the "move more" approach to weight loss was researchers' inability to track calorie output in free-living individuals. Only recently has it become possible to track energy expenditure in a group of participants that modeled ancestral-style living (highly active lifestyles of foraging, hunting, and gathering). Scientists can compare this to another human living an entirely different lifestyle in modern-day America, sitting at a desk filing TPS reports (like our friends in the movie *Office Space*) or spending your days sitting and selling paper at Dunder Mifflin in *The Office* with our friend Michael Scott.

Another barrier used to be the lack of a tool to assess calorie burn or energy expenditure (besides the technology typically used in a metabolic chamber). Evolutionary anthropologists have worked around this issue by using physiologist Nathan Lifson's approach to tracking energy expenditure: the doubly labeled water method, which measures expenditure via carbon dioxide production and is much easier to utilize in free-living environments. Scientists have applied this method to free-living individuals in rural areas of less-developed countries where people live similar lifestyles to our ancestors so that we can compare their metabolisms to those of people living in the modern-day Western world.

For example, a 2008 study from Amy Luke at Loyola University discovered that despite leading completely different lifestyles, women in rural Nigeria had similar energy expenditure to women living in Chicago in a modern urban and likely sedentary environment. Luke also collaborated with Herman Pontzer from Duke University on a study of the Hadza tribe in Tanzania, revealing similar results around their movement levels and energy expenditure in comparison to the expenditure of individuals engaged in habits that are traditionally associated with the Western world.[16]

We also see metabolic constraints with cardiovascular exercise activity. A group of researchers measured total daily energy expenditure in thirty-two adults, split equally between untrained men and women, over a forty-four-week period. The researchers strategically ramped up the volume of training over the study period while also measuring total daily energy intake. Over the trial period, the total daily energy expenditure of the sixteen men decreased, while the total daily energy expenditure of the sixteen women remained the same, indicating that exercise may not have an additive effect on energy expenditure or metabolic rate like we once expected.

None of this is to say that you shouldn't exercise or that movement is for the birds. Walking and resistance training are especially important for sustainable body composition changes and fat loss as well as overall health. The key takeaway here: *you should exercise for the health benefits and to improve your body's response to the food you are eating, not as your sole strategy for weight loss.* You need a blend of nutrition and exercise for optimal results. Excessive exercise or excessive dietary restriction will not necessarily get you to your goals faster.

The key premise from the anthropological data is that metabolism is adaptive when it comes to repeated bouts of energy expenditure. The body has an "energy budget" and will make allocations toward activity or baseline repair. Logically, this energy budgeting makes sense: high activity levels with low amounts of food (a.k.a. energy) would be a perceived stressor for our body because it threatens survival.

If daily energy expenditure can be constrained and increasing exercise volume could reach a point of diminishing returns, this means it's especially important to emphasize our dietary strategies and the implications of energy intake.

It's also important to consider the effect of potential differences in training style on body composition (for example, resistance training versus cardiovascular exercise) and the potential for constraints in metabolism. In most cases when people become frustrated with lack of weight loss, it can be attributed to lacking an appropriate nutritional strategy and failing to pair a nutritional strategy with the correct movement strategy. In other words, the body is choosing to adapt (potentially against our best intentions) to conserve or constrain energy expenditure after repeatedly misaligned diet and exercise attempts.

Before discussing *where* we see these adaptations and viable solutions to address them, it is important to understand what contributes to total daily energy expenditure (TDEE), which is the sum of non-exercise activity (NEAT), thermic effect of food (TEF), exercise activity (EAT), and basal (or resting) metabolic rate. NEAT, EAT, and TEF can change depending on our behaviors, habits, and health history.

- Total daily energy expenditure (TDEE): The total number of calories you burn each day. It is sometimes referred to as your net metabolic rate.

- Non-exercise activity (NEAT): Calories burned from daily activity like walking, chores, playing with your kids, etc.

- Exercise activity (EAT): Calories burned specifically from exercise activity, such as your time in the gym or from your regularly scheduled workout.

- Thermic effect of food (TEF): Calories burned from consumption of food or essentially the cost of eating. Protein has an especially high thermic effect.

- Basal or resting metabolic rate (BMR or RMR): The amount of calories your body burns simply by being alive and completing baseline tasks like breathing and supplying your brain with energy. If you sat on the couch all day long and did nothing but breathe, this would be roughly the number of calories you'd burn.

BMR typically accounts for 50–70% of your daily energy needs. The other components that make up the remaining balance are your non-exercise activity level, exercise activity level, and TEF.

During a prolonged dieting phase or attempts at caloric restriction, we are likely to see a decrease in variable components of energy expenditure such as NEAT, EAT, and TEF. A decrease in TDEE during prolonged dieting is referred to as metabolic adaptation or metabolic compensation (or adaptive thermogenesis in research and academic journal articles). Conversely, in a phase of adding food (also known as a reverse or recovery diet), we are likely to see an increase in TDEE. For otherwise healthy and lean individuals, more food makes the body less "thrifty" about how it uses calories.

This means that in cases of both caloric subtraction and caloric addition, your body will make changes in its utilization of energy and the prevalence of certain hormones to keep you alive. We also see this when the body adapts to phases of calorie excess with diet- and lifestyle-induced disease such as type 2 diabetes. When we intentionally or unintentionally add excessive food, the body adapts to this calorie surplus by storing the calories in fat or muscle tissue, depending on exercise activity and lifestyle factors. If done for too long, this can have serious implications related to an individual's cardiometabolic health and chronic disease risk.

While the tribal or ancestral living examples of indigenous, free-living people addressed largely non-exercise activities such as walking, gathering, and foraging, we also see similar metabolic constraints with cardiovascular exercise activity. The Midwest Exercise Trial looked at the effects of supervised exercise on energy expenditure, energy intake, and body weight. In this trial, non-exercise activity decreased in both men and women. The one limitation of these two examples is that the studies only measured TDEE,[17] not whether the reduction in non-exercise energy expenditure was due to changes in behavior, physiology, or both. Another worthwhile consideration would be examining if similar adaptations would be seen in a group of resistance-trained participants.

This section was not created to suggest that we shouldn't diet or that all exercise attempts are fruitless. It's intended to create awareness and form a foundational understanding of the need for different seasons of nutrition and dieting. From a dietary application standpoint, knowing how many times a person has attempted to "diet" and how dramatically or intensely they've subtracted calories can explain a lot of their frustration with their inability to lose weight. While changes in resting metabolism are possible, time is better spent managing our most controllable variables: nutrition, lifestyle, and movement.

When we zoom in on concerns related to metabolic adaptation, we see that changes in metabolism are usually associated with three factors: The *depth* of a diet, or calorie deficit, is defined by the total number of calories subtracted from your maintenance intake (the amount of energy obtained from food where you can maintain your body weight at your current activity level over an extended period). If you tracked your food for seven days and that amount of food resulted in zero net change to your scale weight, that would be your maintenance intake. If Sally wants to lose weight and stops eating her normal 500-calorie breakfast, this is the depth to which she has reduced her food intake.

The *duration* of the diet is the length of time spent attempting to lose weight during a particular phase of dieting. For example, if Kevin tries to cut calories from his normal maintenance intake by using keto and reducing carbohydrate intake for six months, the duration would be defined by the length of this endeavor—six months, in Kevin's case. Speaking from anecdotal experience, the more extreme the depth and duration of dietary restriction, the harder it is to adhere to the diet or sustain long-term weight loss.

Frequency is the number and severity of previous dietary attempts. It is one of the largest problems in diet culture. Due to the recurring theme of individuals not being able to sustain their weight loss—or, worse yet, regaining more weight than they originally lost—we see repeated attempts to diet or try new fad diets as they emerge. This often compounds the issues. Significant duration and depth paired with frequency creates a recipe for metabolic adaptation.

Not all attempted diets result in a successful calorie deficit; however, all attempted diets put a significant amount of psychological and physiological stress on the body when conducted in an improper fashion. This stress could be from the belief that the diet is a form of self-imposed restraint or restriction, increased exercise activity, or otherwise. So, while the frequency of dieting certainly has physiological effects on the body (which we'll discuss in the section on metabolic adaptation), it has mental effects as well. Stressing "good" and "bad" foods, feelings of shame, difficulty navigating social situations, and self-imposed rules that create rigidity and restriction take a psychological toll on dieters. Failed past diet attempts lead to always seeking the next program, the next diet, or the ever-fleeting quick fix and often looking outside of ourselves instead of within our lives to find the solution to our problems.

With the baseline knowledge of metabolism and seasons of nutrition that you will learn in this book, you can match an appropriate, flexible nutrition strategy to your lifestyle and physiology with fewer hard rules and less stress surrounding the process. You will have a greater understanding of your body's energy and recovery demands and how to shift your program to meet its needs in its current state.

Managing metabolic health and using seasonality with your dieting is crucial for restoring homeostasis or the "status quo" between dietary attempts. This practice allows for multiple successful diets in your lifetime, each with the ability to yield the transformative success you desire. While a rotational or periodized approach to nutrition is rarely implemented in mainstream diet advice, we will explore how to accomplish this feat in the mitigating adaptation section when we discuss more on nutrition and how to eat for your goals.

With repeated dieting without breaks or recovery phases we see:

- A basal metabolic rate that has not recovered and is lower than what it should be relative to the predictive TDEE equations used to assess metabolic rate.
- A non-exercise activity level that is reduced, often subconsciously.
- Exercise activity that is reduced.
- Thermic effect of food that is largely unaffected but is reduced solely based on consuming fewer total calories (remember, the thermic effect of food cannot occur without eating food).

COMPONENTS OF TOTAL DAILY ENERGY EXPENDITURE (TDEE)

NEAT - non-exercise activity thermogenesis

REE - resting energy expenditure

TEF - thermic effect of food

EAT - exercise activity thermogenesis

BMR - basal metabolic rate

NREE - non-resting energy expenditure

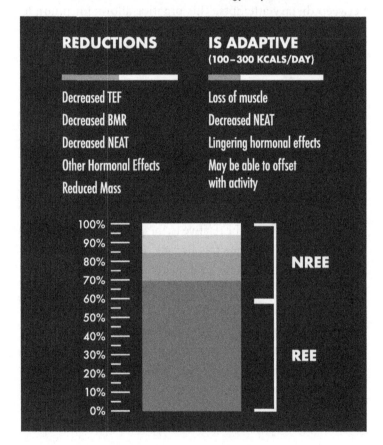

REDUCTIONS

Decreased TEF
Decreased BMR
Decreased NEAT
Other Hormonal Effects
Reduced Mass

IS ADAPTIVE
(100–300 KCALS/DAY)

Loss of muscle
Decreased NEAT
Lingering hormonal effects
May be able to offset with activity

100%
90%
80%
70%
60%
50%
40%
30%
20%
10%
0%

NREE

REE

Metabolism is adaptive. Fat loss is a desired adaptation. People seeking change in their transformation must manage this adaptation. One of the most important variables to consider when managing adaptation is stress, which we'll break down in the following chapter.

STRESS

In modern society, most people treat "stress" like a four-letter word. While often demonized, stress drives adaptation, and some stress is needed to serve as a stimulus for growth or change in the human body. However, excessive stress (whether in amount, duration, or frequency) will lead to delays in reaching physical transformation goals related to appearance, longevity, or performance.

Stress is most often associated with the hormone cortisol. If you follow late-night infomercials too closely, you might attribute cortisol to unwanted body fat or use it as a scapegoat for your transformation goals. The truth is cortisol isn't all bad. We need some cortisol to have morning wakefulness or alertness in challenging situations. Prolonged exposure to stress or chronic stress, on the other hand, can influence your brain and body in unfavorable ways that could potentially hinder your transformation goals.

Cortisol is a steroid hormone (in the glucocorticoid class of corticosteroid hormones) and is synthesized by the adrenal glands in response to stress. It is released in a daily rhythm influenced by our movement and sleep and wake times (sunlight signals the optic nerve in the back of the eye, which helps regulate the central circadian clock).

Cortisol also performs numerous other helpful functions in the body. It is anti-inflammatory, which is why people take prednisone (a synthetic corticosteroid medication) or get cortisone shots when they are in pain and why cortisone creams are used to treat skin conditions like eczema and psoriasis. In addition to being anti-inflammatory, when blood sugar levels drop too low, cortisol is a key player in a process called gluconeogenesis that increases blood sugar and helps provide glucose to cells for energy. Cortisol also assists in digestive processes by triggering gastric acid secretion and assisting in the metabolism of protein, fat, and carbohydrates. It also influences blood pressure.

While we need a baseline amount of cortisol, excess cortisol can be as bad as too little cortisol. The body is collaborative in its allocation of resources when the "emergency" stress response is activated. Think of the body like normal cars on a highway, sharing the road with first responders like police cars and fire trucks. Our hard-wired response uses the same cells, organs, metabolites, and messaging mechanisms that the body uses to manage and maintain our normal non-stress metabolic functions. The body can have dysfunction (accidents) or traffic, depending on the circumstances and external signals that it faces.

Unfortunately, as I write this book in 2021, chronic stress prevails on a daily basis, whether that entails dealing with technology, traffic, coworkers, or the other kids at little Johnny's soccer game. The "fight or flight" system is constantly being triggered, even though these stressors do not pose a danger to our physical survival.

While our human physiology is designed to handle acute bouts of physical stress (such as being hunted down by a predator), it wasn't meant to cope with perpetual psychological and emotional burden that has become a normal part of modern life (such as worrying about paying bills, final exams, or being accessible 24/7 by text, email, or social media). One of the biggest changes in modern society is that *our stressors have been decoupled from movement.* Our prior stressors were largely activity based: hunting, gathering, climbing, carrying, or physically defending ourselves. Those stressors look quite different from defending your inbox, engaging in feisty dialogue on social media, or responding to a confrontational text message.

When considering stress, it is important to understand that in addition to our daily, weekly, or monthly **perceived stressors**, the body is experiencing its own internal stress as a result of our choices. These stressors may include things like glycemic stress, circadian stress, or inflammatory stress, which can manifest as certain health conditions or hormonal and metabolic adaptations as the body attempts to manage the persistent stressor.

In earlier sections, we discussed the idea of energy availability and how a prolonged energy surplus contributes to health complications and metabolic syndrome. Extended energy surplus is one example of **glycemic stress** coupled with inflammatory stress. The term *glycemic* pertains to blood sugar regulation, which is an essential component of health and executive functioning.

Outside of cases of metabolic syndrome and obesity-driven

insulin resistance, the body can also struggle to balance blood sugar when individuals experience chronic stress and excess cortisol production.

Circadian stress refers to the toll or burden the body experiences as a result of conducting our lives in a state of friction relative to our ancestral sleep-wake cycle. Lack of sleep, jet lag, apnea, social jet lag (late nights and weekends), and excessive caffeine consumption can all contribute to stress in this category.

Inflammatory stress can occur in conjunction with glycemic stress as a result of poor food choices and obesity but can also occur in cases of chronic pain, injuries, excessively high-calorie diets (relative to activity levels), metabolic syndrome, and gastrointestinal conditions.

Stress and cortisol are vital during a transformation, so it is essential to have tools in place to self-assess and manage our stress levels and biofeedback—essentially the signs, signals, and symptoms indicative of the body's state of well-being and internal health status. By tracking these markers alongside our nutrition and exercise, we assemble an arsenal of data to understand metabolism, break through plateaus, and achieve lasting success with individualized nutrition.

SELF-ASSESSMENT AND THE TRANSFORMATION FRAME

Perhaps the largest mistake dieters across the world make is embarking on a new plan or program without taking the necessary steps to assess their current health or metabolic status quo. How can you know how to make progress from where you are to where you want to be if you don't know where you are to begin with?

At this stage, working with a qualified professional who understands health, fitness, and nutrition can be helpful. However, not everyone has the ability to work with a coach, so in this section, you will learn tools, tips, and tactics to assess progress, bring awareness to current strengths and weaknesses, course correct any program misalignment, and provide insights for future decision-making.

Before embarking on a new diet or intensifying your exercise program, ask yourself:

- Have you attempted to diet in the last six months? How did that go?
- What sacrifices are you willing to make to your current day-to-day routine to ensure success with this plan?
- What did the duration of your past diets look like?
- How frequently have you attempted different diet or exercise programs?
- When you reduced calories, what was the depth of the reduction?

THE TRANSFORMATION FRAME

Framing the transformation process can be difficult. There are seemingly countless variables to focus on and an abundance of information from books, social media sources, and friends or distant relatives whose input you never asked for. The truth is there are many different ways to achieve your health and fitness or weight-loss goals. However, identifying the best approach requires an understanding of your uniqueness as an individual.

The vast majority of people embark on a fitness or nutrition journey to create changes in their appearance or health. What is often neglected is that the physical outcomes follow the internal physiological workings. We manage our physiology through our habits. We manage our mindset and brain through our perceptions, which also impacts our physiology because the brain governs integral components of human metabolism. Only once we realize this can we begin to permanently shape our physical selves (rather than relying on quick-fix thirty-day changes).

Remember, there is a lot more going on in your body than just the physical stuff you see on the outside. Your body is a biological machine designed to survive famine, cold, and scary stuff coming near your cave with teeth sharper than your finest kitchen cutlery. It is meant to adapt to the physical stuff you throw at it to ensure your survival.

For maximal success in transformation, you can start by taking personal inventory of the three Ps listed below.

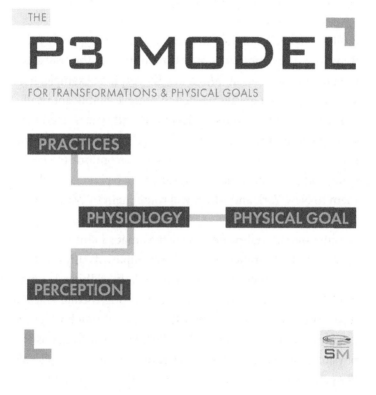

THE

P3 MODEL

FOR TRANSFORMATIONS & PHYSICAL GOALS

PRACTICES

PHYSIOLOGY — **PHYSICAL GOAL**

PERCEPTION

SM

PRACTICES

Transformation practices consist of intentional or unintentional routines, rituals, and regimens that influence the physical and mental state of the body. Some practices are intentional, and others are unintentional. In *Atomic Habits,* author James Clear uses the example of a plane taking off from Los Angeles en route to New York.[18] If the pilot decided to adjust course 3.5 degrees south, the plane's nose would move just a few feet at takeoff. Outside of the cockpit, no one on board would notice the small movement, but the plane would end up in Washington, D.C., instead of New York. This scenario is analogous to the health and fitness journeys of millions of individuals every year.

Positive change requires both patience and the proper practices. Repeating these practices over time improves the trajectory of your transformation. Much like the airplane example, massive change is not always needed to achieve significant results. Sometimes a mere course correction is all that is needed to yield major improvements. The challenging aspect of health and fitness practices is that there are countless options to choose from, and most consumers are unsure which practices will take them to New York and which will route them to Washington.

Specific nutritional protocols such as macro-counting, carb cycling, and intermittent fasting are examples of daily practices or behaviors. Other practices include daily walking, training modalities, animal-based or plant-based eating, meditation, and recovery protocols. Practices are the window through which we can build confidence and self-belief while also making positive physiological changes. Some practices are universally applicable, like getting more sleep. Other practices may vary depending on an individual's lifestyle and health. For example, exercise and a calorie deficit may relieve stress from the body of an overweight type 2 diabetic, but it would compound the problems faced by an overtrained, underfed athlete. You might have a friend who enjoys fasting and plant-based eating, but that might not be the best approach for others. This nuance is often lost in common dietary interventions.

In many cases, this nuance is what is most frustrating about the health, fitness, and nutrition industry. It's nearly impossible to find accurate information around the proper practices due to the overabundance of misinformation and lofty claims. This information overload leads people to adopt practices that are not conducive to their goals and ultimately create physiological changes or adaptations that they never intended—or, worse yet, they quit entirely. Whether these people quit or stick with an approach misaligned to their goals, it often detracts from their progress toward their physical goals. In reality, daily practices can evolve, shift, and grow over time to allow for not only immediate physical gain but lifelong health and fitness.

PERCEPTION

Our perception largely influences our response to chronic stress and the way we view ourselves and food. These perceptions influence the adaptive response that ultimately takes place inside of us—the changes in our physiology. Professors, PhDs, and advocates of stoicism have based their entire careers on the concept of managing our reactions to acute and chronic stress, along with shaping our mindset. The whole concept of adaptive physiology and the neuroendocrine system is to protect us from perceived threats and food scarcity. While our body will likely always perceive a significant physical stressor like a calorie deficit or lack of food as a threat, there are elements of our lives that we can adjust, such as the way we react to things like work stress, family stress, or even the small nuisance of rush hour traffic.

Dr. Carol Dweck defined mindset as a self-perception or "self-theory" that people hold. Believing that you are either "intelligent" or "unintelligent" is a simple example of a mindset. People may also have a mindset related to their personal or professional lives—"I'm a good teacher" or "I'm a bad parent," for example. People can be aware or unaware of their mindsets, but their mindsets can have profound effects on learning achievement, skill acquisition, personal relationships, professional success, and many other dimensions of life.

A study by Alia Crum of Stanford University shows an example of mindset or transformation perceptions in action.[19] This study measured eighty-four female room attendants working in seven different hotels on physiological health variables affected by exercise. It split the housekeepers into groups and gave one group information that might influence their mindset. The other group was not provided with this information.

Those in the informed group were told that the work they did as housekeepers (cleaning hotel rooms) was good exercise and satisfied the surgeon general's recommendations for an active lifestyle. The housekeepers were also provided with examples of how their work was analogous to exercise.

Four weeks after the intervention, the informed group perceived themselves to be getting significantly more exercise than before. As a result, compared with the control group, they showed a decrease in weight, blood pressure, body fat, waist-to-hip ratio, and body mass index. These results support the hypothesis that exercise affects health in part or in whole via the placebo effect. It is also possible that telling the housekeepers they were already active may have resulted in the participants taking part in other healthy behaviors because they identified with taking part in a healthy lifestyle.

An additional look at the placebo effect and the impact of our perception on our physical well-being can be found in a 2002 study from the *New England Journal of Medicine*.[20] In a controlled trial of arthroscopic surgery for osteoarthritis of the knee, a total of 180 patients were randomly assigned to receive arthroscopic debridement, arthroscopic lavage, or placebo surgery. Patients in the placebo group received skin incisions and underwent a simulated debridement without insertion of the arthroscope. Patients and assessors of outcome were blinded to the treatment-group assignment, meaning neither the participants nor the individuals assessing the outcome knew who had received the placebo surgery. The patients were then assessed on a knee-specific pain scale and other markers. The placebo group scored similar to the patients who received the arthroscopic procedure, meaning the outcomes after arthroscopic lavage or arthroscopic debridement were no better than those after a placebo procedure.

As illustrated by the two studies above, our mindset and view of the world play a vital role in both our perception of our well-being and physical markers of well-being. Perception is the glue that integrates practices and physiology because we can utilize practices such as a morning routine, a specific type of exercise, or a specific type of diet that is individualized to a person to make life less stressful.

Remember, given the role of the brain and hypothalamus in the neuroendocrine system, no transformational model would be complete without including an individual's perception of stress.

Here are a few ways to ensure stress isn't getting the best of you in your health and fitness pursuits:

1. Do your best to manage stress through elimination, organization, and simplification.
2. Be more resilient by being less rigid. Bruce Lee once said, "Notice that the stiffest tree is most easily cracked, while the bamboo or willow survives by bending with the wind."
3. Do things that bring you joy.
4. Organize and plan in a manner best suited to your personality.
5. Intentionally schedule downtime.
6. Avoid burning the candle at both ends. For some people, this could mean ending your habit of saying yes to too many obligations or responsibilities. For others, this might be refraining from trying to hit the gym fourteen times per week. Even the most motivated, resilient individuals need to audit their true bandwidth and decide if their choices are serving them.
7. Consider nature walks, yoga, massage, acupuncture, creative therapies (art/music), breathwork, or meditation to help relaxation.
8. Avoid multitasking. Task switching is lethal, and multitasking is a lie. Take small breaks in between tasks.
9. Start a journal or make your own list. Be mindful of what makes you feel better and what makes you feel worse.
10. Connect with others and the community, whether it's pets, family, or other relationships.

Outside of simply managing chronic stress, perception plays a vital role in our relationship with food and relationship with ourselves and our community. In cases of anorexia or bulimia, we see physical and physiological changes as a result of skewed perceptions and poor relationships with food and exercise. This rather extreme illustration shows how perception and practices can negatively influence physiology. Further, it reveals how mindset can ultimately lead someone to intentionally starve themselves and create specific physiological adaptations to metabolism and hormonal health. For most of us, perception starts with basic things like how we view the world and our thoughts on exercise and concepts as "metaphysical" as self-belief and confidence.

PHYSIOLOGY

Physiology is a challenging aspect of the P3 model to influence, largely because it is a consequence of our perception and practices. Unless you are faced with a chronic disease or preexisting medical condition, the truth is your physiology is likely a product of the habits, routines, and rituals that you have established over the course of your lifetime. If you are always over exercising, and under recovering, or under exercising and overeating, your physiology is simply a reflection of your behaviors.

What makes this so difficult is often we think we are doing right by ourselves physically due to the prevalence of misinformation. Sally wants to go to HIIT workouts eight times per week because her friends go and say it is good for weight loss. Sally chooses to not eat carbohydrates for ten days because she saw it on the news or on a magazine cover while she was in the checkout line at the store. Sally now thinks that she has the appropriate practices in place to achieve her desired physical results, but she fails to realize that her selected workout requires carbohydrates and is glycolytic in nature. The level of stress that this restriction imposes on her body leads to physiological changes that are misaligned with her physical goals of being toned and getting ready for her family beach trip.

By relying on the other two Ps, perception and practices, we can influence our physiology and ultimately our physical appearance.

THE PULSE OF YOUR TRANSFORMATION AND P3 APPLIED

Determining your current physiological state and the appropriate daily practices will require significant self-assessment. In this section, we'll discuss tools, methods, and frameworks to determine the best nutrition and exercise approach for you.

FINDING THE PULSE OF YOUR TRANSFORMATION

After coaching clients for over a decade and serving as a mentor for coaches around the globe, I realized that a simple and streamlined intake and assessment process is essential for evaluating the best possible nutrition and training approaches for an individual. Whether you are working with a professional or self-coaching, doing a little bit of upfront work, organization, and checking in can save significant strife over the long haul.

The PULSE of your transformation consists of the following elements:

- Physical goals and objectives
- Understanding key motivators
- Lifestyle
- SHREDS Biofeedback
- Expectations

PHYSICAL GOALS AND OBJECTIVES

Physical goals and objectives might include specific desires around losing weight, dropping a dress size, lowering a percentage of body fat, or developing muscle in your legs or arms. Typically, I recommend picking one goal from a genre of performance, longevity, or body composition. For example, performing better at a sport or for a competition typically requires more food (fuel) and potentially different training or exercise than a body composition goal. A longevity or health-oriented goal might overlap with body composition if losing body fat would improve your overall health status.

UNDERSTANDING KEY MOTIVATORS

No one knows your true underlying motivators like you do. Whether it's feeling more confident, more attractive, or more physically capable, only you know your true desires. Get clear on the why behind your decision to make adjustments to your eating, movement, and lifestyle choices. Ask yourself:

- Why do you have this goal?

- Are you seeking confidence or compensating for another area of life?
- Why is looking good in a bikini important?
- What does more muscle, less fat, or more aesthetically pleasing arms, legs, or abs signify?
- What will life look like after obtaining the stated goal?

LIFESTYLE

One of the more tragic elements of the health and fitness industry is that for so long, dietary approaches have not considered the most basic elements of a person's life. Who cooks your meals? What do you do for work? What type of foods do you have access to? Are you working out at a gym? When do you sleep? How is the quality of your sleep?

Whether it be fat loss, muscle gain, or improved health, sustaining your transformation results requires continued alignment between your lifestyle and the behaviors to achieve and maintain your goal physique.

SHREDS

The SHREDS acronym signifies that we are tracking and gathering information on sleep, hunger, recovery, energy, digestion, and stress baselines. These are important forms of biofeedback indicators that can be used to gauge how well (or how poorly) the body responds to a given set of nutrition and exercise practices. Think of SHREDS as signals and metrics that represent internal health status. This tool will come up in multiple sections because it can be used as both a starting assessment tool and a weekly check-in. Using SHREDS can help inform decision-making about food choices, lifestyle choices, and exercise choices.

SLEEP

Prolonged dieting can impact sleep duration and quality. Compromised sleep can also influence hormone production, insulin sensitivity, and willpower. Consider both sleep quality (how rested do you feel?) and sleep quantity (how many hours did you sleep?).

HUNGER

Nobody likes being hungry all the time. While some hunger is bound to occur during a diet phase or season of restricted calorie intake, appetite management is crucial for creating a sustainable program. Ask yourself:

- On a scale of 1 to 10, how is your hunger?
- When are you most hungry vs. least hungry?

In sections that follow, we'll discuss managing hunger using protein and fiber, along with a few other satiety tips and tricks.

RECOVERY

Training and nutrition protocols must be aligned to allow for ample recovery from exercise. Poor recovery will often result in lackluster performance and exercise effort in subsequent sessions, leading to less progress in the overall transformation. To assess your recovery, consider soreness, training motivation, progressive overload, and performance.

ENERGY

Chronic dieting can induce fatigue and lethargy, and zap energy. Managing energy and blood sugar levels is vital for a successful diet phase.

DIGESTION

Food is more than the flavors we taste. Our food provides fuel for our cells and requires ample effort from our gastrointestinal tract to not only assimilate and absorb nutrients but also to excrete food waste and detoxify our bodies. When looking at digestive health, it is important to consider both the quality and quantity of bowel movements. Regular trips to the toilet should be part of your day-to-day routine. If you are not experiencing regular and healthy bowel movements (a quick search for a "bristol stool chart" online can be an easy way to assess this), this should be a consideration prior to embarking on a more deliberate attempt at fat loss and calorie restriction. While it is possible to tackle both digestive health and body recomposition, it is imperative to remember that dieting in and of itself is a stressor contributing to a catabolic physiological state and that gastrointestinal issues can often have a strong stress component.

STRESS

In the twenty-first century, life is ripe with stressful experiences that look significantly different from those of our paleolithic ancestors. Not only can our lifestyles induce stress, but our food and exercise habits also can either impose or alleviate stress on the body. Stress can be either acute or chronic and can be caused by lifestyle or protocols.

EXPECTATIONS

Results don't happen overnight. The thirty-day challenges and eight-minute ab blasts often overpromise and underdeliver when it comes to tangible transformation progress. We get frustrated due to miscommunication, unfulfilled expectations, and lack of progress, which often manifests as an inability to maintain consistency in the transformation. If you've previously fallen victim to the marketing hype and gimmicky transformation approaches, understand these programs are ripe with false promises.

Rather than having outcome-oriented expectations, develop a clear picture of action-oriented expectations that can be defined as keeping promises to yourself. Personal integrity on a daily and weekly basis will create undeniable momentum and progress toward your goals. You can start building integrity by going to sleep on time, drinking more water, or going for a walk each day. Ask yourself:

- What will you do to ensure you make nutrition decisions aligned with your goals?
- Do you have a training program? How often will you exercise?
- How will you plan, schedule, and prepare to successfully follow your program?
- What will you do if you fall off track briefly?

PULSE SUMMARIZED

By getting a thorough PULSE or understanding of your starting metrics, you can begin to make evaluations on important considerations such as metabolic status, stress, health, and diet history to determine the most realistic and sustainable approach moving forward.

TRANSFORMATION TOOLS FOR MANAGING METABOLISM

What gets lost in life, but *especially* in the fitness industry, is that every season is one of becoming but not always one of blooming. This idea is especially relevant during the typical New Year "season of resolutions."

Don't get me wrong—some of the best things in life come as a result of seasons. And no, I'm not talking about pumpkin spice or peppermint mocha coffee. But not every season is one where you should be dieting or peaking for an event or competition. While nutritional periodization has made some headway, as have reverse diets, the unfortunate truth is that 95% of diets fail, based on dietary rebound statistics.

Worthwhile accomplishments are nearly always defined by seasons or cycles. Olympic athletes organize their training over four years to precisely peak at the Olympics. Your favorite sports stars have in-season games or competitions, and off-season preparation. Your favorite music artists generally are not on tour year round multiple years in a row. They spend time recording, preparing, and refining their art to create the best possible product when they are "in season" or on stage.

The concept of seasonality with training and nutrition is not a recent discovery, but the ideas have not always reached mainstream consumers. In bodybuilding, Olympic weight-lifting, and other specific sports, coaches have used a concept called periodization, which is the strategy that goes into creating various phases of preparation en route to a goal. Periodization could be a plan used for an athletic pursuit or an appearance-related goal. In my coaching, and for the purposes of this book, I created three distinct phases to describe the most popular pursuits when it comes to nutrition or diet strategy. These are the build, burn, and break "seasons" of nutrition.

The *build* season can be used to build recovery bandwidth and restore your body's physiological function. It is not always just about adding calories, but reverse diets or periods of time spent *not* dieting do fit well here, as do deliberate attempts to build muscle, which requires eating slightly more food.

A *break* can be as simple as a rest day, de-load, refeed, or temporary pause in physiological stress on the body. Whether this is a literal vacation or a short break in your diet or intense training to take a few days off from the gym or eat a bit more food, breaks serve as a way to ease the physiological stress placed on the body.

The *burn* phase sounds sexy to anyone seeking fat loss, but the meaning here is that we are burning through our physiological bandwidth. This would include exercising profusely while undereating and experiencing transient changes or downregulations in hormones. A little "burn phase" can be good, but a nonstop attempt at achieving a calorie deficit for years on end is not a wise move for your long-term health and fitness goals. By cycling "break" and "build" phases in with your "burn" phases, you have a greater likelihood of resilience from both a physiological and a psychological perspective. Burn sounds like it might only apply to a pursuit at fat burning, but it can also apply to intense training for a competition, race, or meet. A great example here is something like the CrossFit Open, which is an intense process even for recreational athletes and should be viewed as a block of time where the body is under significantly more stress from the demands of training and intense exercise.

Each phase or season is a lever. When you pull the right lever, you move closer to the end result you are looking to achieve while maintaining optimal health in the process. Most people will need to spend balanced amounts of time between phases. So if you choose to diet for four months, you will also likely need to spend some time where you incorporate breaks or build phases in order to mitigate some of the symptoms of metabolic adaptation discussed in prior chapters.

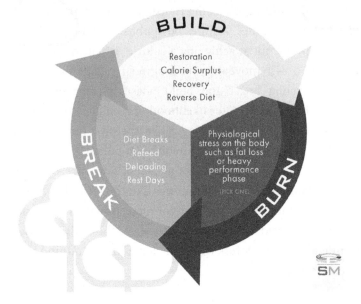

SEASONS OF NUTRITION
NUTRITIONAL PERIODIZATION SIMPLIFIED...

BUILD

Restoration
Calorie Surplus
Recovery
Reverse Diet

BREAK

Diet Breaks
Refeed
Deloading
Rest Days

BURN

Physiological
stress on the body
such as fat loss
or heavy
performance
phase

(PICK ONE)

SM

MANAGING METABOLISM FOR SUSTAINABLE CHANGES

Using the seasons of nutrition and the SHREDS model allows us to make better daily, weekly, and monthly decisions for our body. But you might wonder what exactly you should change, adjust, or modify as a result of this information. This confusion is precisely why I created a check-in checklist using what I call the ten transformation toggles or transformation toolkit. By strategically using the ten toggles, we can streamline our transformation efforts, improve our biofeedback, and move ourselves closer to our physical goals. The ten toggles are the activities that define our daily practices within the P3 model. You could think of them as your *transformation toolkit*.

THE TEN TRANSFORMATION TOGGLES IN YOUR TRANSFORMATION TOOLKIT

1. SLEEP

Though the other items in this list appear in no particular order, I intentionally placed sleep in the top spot. Sleep primes the body via recovery, improves insulin sensitivity, and is essential for hormone production. Often, plateaus in fat loss or muscle building can be traced back to inadequate sleep and recovery. Sleep is one of the most underrated facets of improving health and body composition in that until recently, it wasn't an area that received much marketing attention. Most people need to add or improve their sleep to move closer to their fitness goals. Starting with an evening routine, keeping your room cool and dark, and minimizing technology before bed can all help to improve sleep quality. Aim to include seven or more hours of quality sleep in the pursuit of any transformation goal. There's not one magic number for everyone. Start with this minimum as a suggested baseline and work to find your sweet spot from there. Note: hours asleep and hours in bed are not the same! You will likely need more than seven hours in bed to achieve seven hours of sleep.

Downsides of chronic sleep restriction:

- Decreases testosterone
- Decreases growth hormone
- Increases ghrelin
- Decreases leptin
- Increases cortisol
- Decreases thyroid function
- Decreases insulin sensitivity

As illustrated above, lack of sleep also causes many of the same adaptations we see from chronic dieting. If you combine the two, you are creating a recipe for disaster in that many of the hormones above are responsible for retaining lean muscle, losing fat, and improving our receptivity, partitioning, and effective utilization of the nutrients that we eat.

2. NON-EXERCISE ACTIVITY

One of the perks of non-exercise activity (or movement outside the gym) is that it burns calories without the nervous system stress or stimulation that comes as a part of intense exercise. Walking has been shown to improve insulin sensitivity, digestion, and other key markers of health. This non-exercise activity is also a crucial component of total daily energy expenditure (as explained in earlier sections detailing the science of metabolism and energy output). Other examples of non-exercise activity include chores, play, fidgeting, and other types of movement outside of your training sessions.

Interrupting prolonged sitting with brief bouts of light walking attenuates post-meal glucose responses, insulin levels, and triglycerides in type 2 diabetes.[21] Fifty to seventy minutes of walking three days per week can lower visceral fat and abdominal fat and improve glucose levels and inflammatory markers.[22] In fact, regular activity (not just exercise or resistance training) has such a potent effect on health that some have suggested it could be used as an alternative or adjunct to drug therapy. Regular walking leads to positive changes in resting heart rate, body fat, total cholesterol, depression, and quality of life for physical functioning.[23]

3. STRESS MANAGEMENT

Most individuals have heard the phrase "you can't pour from an empty cup," yet in modern society, it is rare to see a deliberate effort to focus on recovery-centric activities that fill our proverbial cup. Whether you prefer meditation, breathwork, journaling, or talking through issues with a confidant, stress management helps to ensure proper cortisol patterns and the health of our brain-adrenal axis. When you fail to manage stress, it can influence daily dietary decisions and the ability to achieve quality sleep. The key is not so much the activity itself but the ability of that chosen activity to bring you back to the present moment. To quote the old adage and the wise sensei Master Oogway from the children's movie *Kung Fu Panda*, "Yesterday is history, tomorrow is a mystery, but today is a gift. That is why it is called the present."[24]

Each flavor of stress management may have varying effects depending on the chosen activity, the duration of the activity, and your unique enjoyment and appreciation of the activity. When looking at stress management techniques, music interventions may have positive effects on physiological signs of stress like heart rate and blood pressure, as well as on hormone levels.[25] Other art-related therapies include drawing, sketching, dance movement therapy, and drama therapy.

In addition, individuals can also benefit from alternative stress management techniques such as progressive muscle relaxation and mindfulness, which help reduce emotional exhaustion, depression, anxiety, and occupational stress.[26]

Another stress management tactic is time in nature. While time outside is included for its obvious benefits for vitamin D synthesis, studies of wilderness-like sites compared to indoor exercise facilities or parks also show a greater reduction in salivary cortisol and perceived stress. As little as ten to twenty minutes and up to fifty minutes of sitting or walking in a diverse array of natural settings has significant positive impacts on key psychological and physiological markers when contrasted with equal durations spent in urbanized settings.[27]

4. CALORIE ALLOTMENT

While a calorie from a Twinkie or a Pop-Tart does not provide the same level of micronutrient density as a calorie provided from protein-rich wild game, pasture-raised eggs, vegetables, or fruit, we still need to be mindful of the role of energy balance and the stimuli that certain foods provide our body. Plateaus in weight loss or training performance can often be traced back to total energy intake across weeks, months, or years.

5. MACRONUTRIENT ALLOCATION

Macronutrients each have their own unique purpose in overall health. We need essential amino acids for muscular development and recovery, while essential fats are beneficial for brain health and other components of longevity (see earlier chapters for the discussion of the unique roles and importance of each nutrient).

6. MICRONUTRIENTS, HYDRATION, AND FIBER

Vitamins, minerals, and water are often overlooked when it comes to fad diets or chronic dieting decisions. These nutrient superheroes are needed for essential processes and reactions throughout the body. We need zinc, selenium, and iodine for thyroid health, while vitamin D has hormone-like effects and acts on receptors throughout our body. These are just a few essential nutrients that influence our quality of life, fitness, and physique aspirations. All too often, fad approaches fail to account for these pivotal transformation variables.

7. EATING CHRONOLOGY

Eating chronology is a scientific way of talking about the timing of your meals or food consumption (e.g., time-restricted eating or intermittent fasting). Time-restricted eating can be used to improve adherence, create a calorie deficit, or give the GI tract a break from frequent meals and digestive burden. This toggle is simply a tool, not a requirement for progress, despite what many autophagy zealots will tell you. Nutrition can also be structured in a way to enhance sleep quality and workout recovery. Nutrient timing or chrono-nutrition isn't always our biggest consideration, but it can be a helpful way to manage individual client cases. Micromanaging meal timing is likely a bad idea if you have a poor relationship with food or a prior history of restriction or eating disorder diagnosis. For more on eating chronology, consider seeking out research or books specific to circadian biology and eating.

Time-restricted eating does not outweigh variables like energy balance, food quality, portion control, and energy expenditure. However, it can be a useful intervention for improving cardiometabolic health when also accounting for other variables in our checklist, such as calories, macronutrients like protein, micronutrient density, exercise, and sleep.

8. FOOD GROUP ELIMINATION

Certain camps of dieters believe that eliminating entire food types is a surefire way to improve health. It also directly reduces calorie consumption, which can be the driving force in individuals seeing results. Note that just because something is gluten-free or vegan doesn't mean it's healthy. Often individuals become "starchans" as opposed to actually eating predominantly plant-based foods like vegetables. Food group elimination is merely a tool for individuals who require this level of specificity or face particular challenges related to digestion or tolerability of specific food groups.

9. EXERCISE ACTIVITY

While individuals typically over-rely on exercise activity to create energy balance or a caloric deficit, it is still a very important component of a transformation and overall health. It's also key for weight maintenance after weight loss. Exercise activity, especially in the form of resistance training, is a powerful tool for muscle building and thwarting degenerative conditions such as osteoporosis and osteopenia. Muscle not only equips us with the strength for daily activities but also serves as an endocrine organ in its own right, positively signaling tissues, glands, and organs across the body.

10. RELATIONSHIPS AND COMMUNITY

You might not expect to see these terms on a list geared toward producing an optimal physical transformation, but relationships and community are key factors of longevity and overall health. Some researchers posit that loneliness is as detrimental as smoking fifteen cigarettes per day.

In a detailed examination in Italy, researchers from the *European Journal of Psychology* found that satisfying social ties with friends and family members, together with an active socially oriented lifestyle, seem to contribute to the promotion of mental health during the adult lifespan.[28] This community component is illustrated in three of the nine tenets of blue zones developed by Dan Buettner and in research in the *American Journal of Lifestyle Medicine*.[29] These three tenets are belonging, the idea of "the right tribe" or moais (groups of five friends that help to cultivate, foster, and encourage healthy behaviors), and putting loved ones first. It is not uncommon for elders to spend their final years at home with their younger family members, which not only improves their longevity but seems to create positive health benefits for young children along with the benefits of passing down wisdom across generations. While some aspects of the "blue zone" research have been called into question, the community or tribal aspect of longevity is supported by a substantial evidence base (like the studies in the *European Journal of Psychology*), while also being in alignment with our ancestral practices as humans.

These community and connection-based health benefits are not limited to humans either. Studies have shown that pets can provide socioemotional benefits for children via stress buffering.[30] In practical terms, this connection means less perceived stress and lower cortisol production—a great combination for anyone looking to improve their health, longevity, and body composition.

The power of relationships in transformations extends to our relationships with food, exercise, and even ourselves. Adopting a flexible, growth-oriented mindset can help bolster your approach to not only health and fitness but other obstacles in life as well.

BONUS TOOL

Once again an unconventional but necessary item to include in this book is time outside. Time in nature or time outdoors is a great way to engage the parasympathetic nervous system, get some extra vitamin D, and increase non-exercise activity energy expenditure. Unfortunately, due to our current infrastructure and nature of work, most individuals do not spend enough time outside, leaving 40% of adults deficient in vitamin D. As mentioned in the stress management toggle, time in nature has the ability to influence both perceived stress and the physiological stress response in human participants.

PART 2

HOW TO EAT

Depending on who you ask, you might hear that eggs are bad for cholesterol, coffee dehydrates you, and plants are either the best or worst thing ever. In fact, the evening before writing this chapter, I stumbled upon an Instagram account where the entire diet consisted of bone marrow, liver, whole eggs, and beef tartar. Every year countless coaches, doctors, celebrities, and media personnel will tell you that there's one best way to eat based on research on humans, animals, a petri dish, or otherwise. While being eggless, plantless, carbless, or meatless may work for some, it doesn't necessarily mean you need to do the same. Nutrition is ripe with nuance—arguably more than any other field. Some Asian cultures have nearly 85% carbohydrates in their diet (from things like rice, bread, potatoes, fruit, vegetables, and pastas or other grain), whereas in Mediterranean cultures and diets, you might find as high as 40% of calories derived from fat (in foods such as oils, butters, meat, egg yolks, nuts, and seeds).

Between this dietary dichotomy and after consuming a significant amount of acronym alphabet soup in this book, you might be wondering what to eat or how to eat based on these tools, methods, models, and frameworks. While we will cover some specific eating styles and strategies, the most important considerations for a successful attempt at fat loss, muscle gain, or body recomposition include eating for present and future fuel (the energy you need for your activity level) and present and future fullness (satiety).

PRESENT AND FUTURE FUEL

One way to think of individual nutrition needs is to plan to eat for what you just did or are about to do. For example, carbohydrates are largely activity-dependent, aside from our liver and brain's baseline need for glucose (the exception being when ketones are the primary energy source on a ketogenic diet). You can determine your energy needs by keeping a seven-day food log and tracking your weight and calorie intake to see if you are maintaining, losing, or gaining weight on your current intake. You can also use TDEE equations or BMR calculators like the "Katch-McArdle" equation if you know your lean body mass. Others use tools like the Mifflin-St Jeor Equation, which can be found easily online. An easier, less math-intensive way to evaluate your TDEE or maintenance calorie intake is to keep a seven-day food log and track your bodyweight. If you maintain your weight, then your caloric intake matches your current expenditure over the seven days. If you gain weight, you are eating more calories or energy than you are burning. If you lose weight, the opposite is true.

When modifying your nutrition or setting starting nutrition goals, set protein first, shooting for 0.8 grams to 1 gram of protein per pound of body weight. Carbs and fats are dependent on a few factors. For serious fitness enthusiasts or bodybuilders, consider raising this protein amount to 1.2 grams per pound (or even 1.5 grams) as needed to promote recovery, as long as your digestion permits. You may need a higher ratio of carbohydrates to fats if you participate in high levels of carbohydrate-demanding activities (also known as glycolytic activity), such as sprinting and weightlifting, or high levels of daily non-exercise activity, or if you have already obtained a lower body fat level and you need to support your performance.

Other reasons for exchanging carbohydrates for fat or vice versa include personal preference and if it helps you to have more stable energy levels without crashes or brain fog. Factors that signify you might do better on less carbs and more fat are largely based on activity levels and personal preference. For example, if you are sedentary or walking is your only form of exercise you *might* benefit from a slightly more fat-dominant diet. You might include fats over carbs if they help manage your appetite or if eating a higher-carb diet leads to post-meal energy crashes. If you are overweight or obese, there is a chance that weight gain has promoted some degree of insulin resistance. While simply controlling calories and portions can begin to address this issue, often controlling carbohydrates can stabilize energy levels and improve your response to meals. Regardless of your current weight or body composition, consider how you feel and your quality of life when you're eating this way. This change takes time and experimentation, so don't worry about it being perfect on the first attempt.

PRESENT AND FUTURE FULLNESS

Another way to individualize nutrition is through finding foods (and the right amounts of foods) that provide satiety during and between meals. Typically, we accomplish this satiety or fullness primarily through protein, water, and fiber intake, along with requisite dietary carbohydrate and fat for our activity level. Note that some people find fat to be more satiating, while others both enjoy and feel full from eating carbohydrates. However, the starting point for present and future fullness begins with protein, water, and fiber. These "ingredients" are key drivers of feelings of fullness and blood glucose stabilization.

Considerations around fullness and satiety often tie back to the concept of volumetrics. Certain foods are more voluminous and filling at a lower calorie total—i.e., vegetables, oatmeal, and other foods with higher water and fiber content. For example, 150 calories of oat bran, 100 calories of raspberries, two whole eggs plus 100 calories of egg whites, and a cup of spinach cooked in would yield well over 10 grams of fiber and 30 grams of protein, along with a substantial amount of "food volume," resulting in more fullness compared to, say, 450 calories from pre-packaged snack foods.

With these two concepts in mind, we can begin to tailor food intake to the individual. In addition to these two key themes, there are subcomponents or categories of dietary success that I call the five Ms: managing appetite, mitigating adaptation, maximizing adherence, minding your micronutrients, and maximizing absorption and assimilation. As a "bonus M" for athletes, remember to match your fuel intake to the activity as I mentioned earlier in the macronutrients section of this book.

MANAGING APPETITE

Few people like feeling hungry on a daily basis. One of the most challenging aspects of dieting is that in subtracting calories to lose weight, we often trigger substantial feelings of hunger and cravings. Conventional diet models typically place restriction first and foremost, above foundational nutrition needs or satiety and fullness.

In research, the hierarchy for macronutrient-induced satiety, or most satiating per unit efficiency, is similar to that observed for diet-induced thermogenesis (DIT): protein is the most satiating macronutrient followed by carbohydrates and fat, which is least satiating.[31]

Note that while these latter two do not necessarily provide the majority of our satiety, they often provide the bulk of our calories in terms of total daily energy intake. While preference for fat or carbohydrate may vary person to person, the research is clear that protein and fiber are the proverbial kings and queens for appetite management.

PROTEIN

Ever have a large portion of steak, chicken, or fish or an omelet where you felt full for hours, or even the rest of the day? This is protein serving up satiety at its finest. Not to mention, small shifts such as shifting protein intake from 10% of calories to 30% of calorie intake can boost metabolic rate, increase fat oxidation, and increase satiety.[32]

Researchers at the University of Kansas Medical Center used fMRIs and found that when subjects added dietary protein to their first meal of the day, it decreased signals in the brain that stimulate appetite and lead to overeating.[33] Sustained satiety is a key component to induce a negative energy balance and to promote weight loss. An ideal weight-loss strategy would promote satiety and maintain basal metabolic rates despite a negative energy balance and reduction in fat-free mass. The challenging aspect of the science of satiety is that it is multi-factorial and influenced by many components, including but not limited to the endocrine system, the cognitive and neural systems, and the gastrointestinal system.

Vast amounts of experimental and real-world research have revealed that increasing the protein composition of the diet without changing net energy can lead to enhanced feelings of satiety or fullness.[34] Potential underlying mechanisms include diet-induced thermogenesis[35] and gastrointestinal hormonal signaling.[36]

Randomized trials of high-protein diets on weight management provide evidence that these types of higher-protein protocols or eating styles can help sustain longer-term weight loss[37] and potentially aid future weight maintenance.[38]

When studied in a laboratory setting, the satiating effects of high-protein foods or meals have been compared to equal-calorie but lower-protein counterparts. These studies typically utilize a "preload" methodology, basing the measure of satiety on a subjective rating after protein consumption where participants rate their appetite and/or food intake. A hefty amount of these types of studies indicate that high protein foods deliver better satiety than energy matched foods with lower levels of protein.[39]

In general, increased satiety has been observed after meals with a protein content in the range of 25% to 81%, and this is a must for weight loss.[40] Across the broad scope of research and evidence, we can see that protein is paramount, and not just for those looking to build new slabs of muscle but also for those looking to manage their appetite and adhere to a diet for weight loss.

Simply put, you can't pass on protein if you are looking for optimal appetite management and a sustainable approach to body transformation. Research conducted by the US Military and cited in *The Journal of Nutrition* found that despite dogmatic beliefs that protein is a threat to longevity, data suggests quite the opposite. Higher-protein diets are associated with lower BMI, lower levels of visceral fat, and an improved cholesterol profile compared to protein intakes at the recommended dietary allowance levels (the RDA for protein is a lower intake).[41] The paramount importance of protein intake doesn't dissipate with age either. Research from Ohio State University indicated that people who didn't eat enough protein were also less likely to get sufficient amounts of micronutrients. The participants in this study, published in *The Journal of Nutrition, Health & Aging,* were ages fifty-one and up, and 46% of the oldest participants did not consume enough protein on a regular basis.[42] While many of you reading this may not be celebrating the half-century mark just yet, this data supports the notion that protein is pivotal throughout the lifespan. So, don't just leave the protein for Arnold Schwarzenegger and his bodybuilding descendants. Prioritize putting protein on your plate even if your sights and your goals are not set on the "Olympia" bodybuilding stage.

FIBER

Generally speaking, dietary fiber is the edible parts of plants or similar carbohydrates that are resistant to digestion and absorption in the small intestine. Dietary fiber can be separated into many different factions. Most simply it is often divided into soluble and insoluble fiber, but more specific groups include arabinoxylan, inulin, pectin, bran, cellulose, β-glucan, and resistant starch.[43] Compared with the digestible carbohydrates, starch, and sugars, fiber has a low energy density in terms of calorie content and may have an attenuating effect on appetite.

Fiber typically comes from plant foods, complete with a unique blend of bioactive components including resistant starches, vitamins, minerals, phytochemicals, and antioxidants. As a result, fiber comes with a host of health benefits, with recent studies supporting an inverse relationship between dietary fiber and the development of several types of cancers, including colorectal, small intestine, oral, larynx, and breast. Aside from the health benefits of fiber, getting fiber from your daily food choices can help make dietary decisions, calorie control, and energy balance easier through appetite management.

Dietary fiber may regulate appetite through a few different mechanisms, the first being physical effects through forming viscous gels. In studies using gel-forming fibers, researchers have seen notable effects on appetite suppression, glucose tolerance, and inflammatory markers.[44] A few examples of gel-forming soluble fiber are psyllium husk, oats, barley, shiitake mushrooms, legumes, and nuts.

The second mechanistic effect of dietary fiber is the production of short-chain fatty acids (SCFAs), which are the main metabolites produced in the colon by bacterial fermentation of dietary fibers and resistant starch.[45] The SCFAs acetate, propionate, and butyrate are the main metabolites produced in the colon by bacterial fermentation of dietary fibers and resistant starch. SCFAs also seem to help with appetite regulation via action on the brain. Studies show effects on several neural functions, such as modulating the signaling triggered by the ghrelin receptor (a receptor for hunger-promoting hormones) and contributing to appetite control, as well as potential sleep and circadian rhythm benefits, which further contribute to overall health and body composition benefits.[46] Foods with SCFA potential include oats, barley, shiitake mushrooms, legumes, nuts, onions, garlic, Jerusalem artichoke, chicory root, green bananas and plantains, leeks, apples, and asparagus. Starches like rice and potatoes that have been cooked and subsequently cooled develop some degree of resistant starch, which falls into this category as well.

Another positive trait of dietary fiber is it is often densely concentrated in foods that also contain water, which helps contribute to appetite regulation and satiety.

WATER

In years of handling a vast array of client cases, I've lost count of the amount of times that a "hungry client" was just thirsty or potentially missing some of our key protein and fiber strategies outlined above. While the exact mechanisms of how water impacts appetite regulation are less clearly established, it makes sense that a dry mouth or empty belly would only contribute to "wanting more" at your next meal. In a 2018 study of healthy young adults, pre-meal water consumption led to a significant reduction in meal energy (calorie) intake, suggesting that pre-meal water consumption may be an effective weight control strategy.[47]

How much water? A 2015 study looked at 350–500ml of water consumption and its effect on subsequent meal calorie consumption in non-obese males. This study demonstrated that consumption of just over 500ml of water thirty minutes prior to a meal reduced the calorie intake at the next meal across study participants. This might be an effective strategy to suppress energy intake and possibly assist with weight management.[48]

Will any beverage do the trick? Not quite. For adults, a systematic review of water consumption and energy intake found reasonable agreement among a number of single-meal studies that replacing water with sugar-sweetened beverages will actually increase your energy intake, so go for water or a non-calorie-containing beverage of choice.[49]

During your next meal or diet phase, consider trying this out for yourself. Not only does water and adequate hydration have a host of health benefits, but you will also potentially consume a lower amount of calories, which is a valuable energy-management and dietary-adherence tool.

Think of water, protein, and fiber as tools for calorie displacement. Imagine the scenario of filling a bathtub. Most tubs can fit a specific volume of water before overflowing. Other objects that take up space, like a human body, can also influence the height of the water in the tub. Generally, the water, protein, and fiber we consume can help displace other calorie-dense food choices that would potentially make it harder to sustain or achieve a calorie deficit.

ATTENTIVE EATING AND EATING PACE

Despite contrary belief, there's more to managing appetite than what goes into your mouth. How we eat can also go a long way in supporting successful improvements to nutrition and body composition. While it is certain that we can achieve health improvements by moving away from the standard American diet choices, decisions like eating pace and distracted eating also influence appetite and satiety.

Have you ever personally powered down a meal in a matter of minutes or witnessed a friend power shovel their way to the clean plate club? Or frantically raced your siblings to the dinner table to scarf down food before someone can steal your serving? Or tried to slam a snack between work meetings and conference calls, or in the after-school pick-up line? When it comes to eating pace, individuals who consume the same calorie content in a meal can have varying post-meal responses in terms of appetite control and subsequent consumption.

In one particular study, two groups were given 600-calorie meals. One group consumed their meals in six minutes, whereas the other group spent twenty-four minutes consuming their meals. The hunger hormone ghrelin (more on this in our adaptation section) was suppressed longer for the twenty-four-minute meal group and appetite was also rated lower. The group that took longer to consume their meal also consumed 25% fewer calories at their next snack, which was three hours after the meal (calorie content of that snack was not controlled by the study, so participants could eat as much or as little as they felt like).[50]

In addition to eating pace, an emphasis also must be placed on focused or attentive eating. In a systematic review, by Robinson, et al., researchers found that attentive eating is likely to influence food intake and could serve as a novel approach to weight loss even without calorie counting because of its ability to reduce the likelihood of overeating at a given meal or during a given day.[51] This makes it a fantastic strategy for anyone trying to improve their health and body composition because regardless of your personal preferences or nutritional beliefs, attentive eating can be used to keep you on track.

MITIGATE ADAPTATION

While managing appetite is essential for achieving a calorie deficit, a delicate balance exists when manipulating our body's energy availability and calorie intake. Further, adherence and appetite are managed meal by meal, and adaptation is managed by signaling the brain and body through food availability or varying calorie totals over time. This signals that energy demands are met, and there are no imminent threats to our survival or well-being (as illustrated in the adaptive physiology section). In other words, dieting certainly isn't a race to the bottom or a game of nutritional limbo, and more importantly, we shouldn't misuse the aforementioned appetite management strategies to perpetually undereat.

The body's sensitivity to energy manipulation rears its head both in terms of hormonal or endocrine adaptations to dieting as well as the effect of weight loss on metabolic rate and total daily energy expenditure. Research describes this process more specifically as energy restriction being accompanied by changes in circulating hormones, mitochondrial efficiency, and energy expenditure that serve to minimize the energy deficit, attenuate weight loss, and promote weight regain.[52]

Hypocaloric diets, where individuals eat significantly below their maintenance calorie intake, induce a number of adaptations that serve to prevent further weight loss and conserve energy. It is likely that the degree to which these adaptations occur is directly related to the amount of calorie restriction or energy deficit (remember the depth, duration, and frequency of diets mentioned in past chapters). For example, studies have observed that fasting, regardless of adipose status, drops leptin levels a very large amount very quickly (60–500% within a three-day fast).[53] These hormonal and metabolic adaptations and why they happen are further explained in the section that follows.

HORMONAL AND METABOLIC ADAPTATIONS TO DIETING

While adaptive physiology can be a gift in many respects, and it works to our advantage to survive in difficult conditions or environments, it can also create additional challenges and friction when pursuing fat loss or body recomposition. A number of hormones play prominent roles in the regulation of body composition, energy intake, and energy expenditure. First, we'll learn the power of these hormones, and then, we'll discuss how to manage them effectively during a diet phase. Some of these hormones are thyroid hormone, leptin, insulin, ghrelin, cortisol, and testosterone.

The hormones of the thyroid gland, particularly triiodothyronine (T3), play an important and direct role in regulating metabolic rate. Increases in circulating thyroid hormones are associated with an increase in the metabolic rate, whereas lowered thyroid levels result in decreased thermogenesis and overall metabolic rate.[54] Many equate thyroid hormone to your metabolic gas pedal because with less thyroid hormone, we burn less energy and generate less heat.

Leptin, synthesized primarily in cells specialized for the storage of fat, functions as an indicator of both short- and long-term energy availability. Short-term energy restriction and being leaner (holding or maintaining a lower body fat percentage) are associated with decreases in circulating leptin. Additionally, higher concentrations of leptin are associated with increased satiety and energy expenditure.[55]

Insulin, an anabolic (building) and anti-catabolic (preservation) hormone, plays a pivotal role in mitigating muscle protein breakdown[56] and regulating the metabolism of macronutrients. Insulin is another signal indicative of levels of body fat.[57] Much like the physiological communication from leptin, high levels of insulin deliver a message of energy availability and are associated with an effect on appetite management (also referred to as an anorexigenic effect).

The yin to leptin and insulin's yang is the hunger hormone ghrelin, which functions to stimulate appetite and food intake and has been shown to increase with fasting and decrease after feeding.[58] Insulin makes sure that we are storing the fuel we consume in the appropriate gas tank, whether that be the muscle tank or the fat tank. With less food coming in during times of intense dieting, we have a lower signal to store energy, and we likely store less fuel in muscle tissue or fat.

Another anabolic, anti-catabolic, but also androgenic hormone is testosterone. Testosterone is often associated with macho behavior, muscularity, or virility, but all humans have testosterone, and it plays an important role in the amount of muscle we are able to build or synthesize. Testosterone also plays a role in fertility and sex drive. It makes sense that with less food or perceived safety and energy in our environment, we downregulate levels of this hormone to preserve energy levels and also downregulate reproductive efforts and desires. But muscle building and fertility are not the only way testosterone plays a role in body composition. Testosterone may also play a role in regulating body fat levels.[59] *Changes in fat mass have been inversely correlated with testosterone levels, and it has been suggested that testosterone may quash the creation of new body fat.*[60] Therefore, for the best results possible, we need to periodically intervene to thwart the reduction of testosterone during an attempt at fat loss or diet phase.

Last but not least is cortisol. Often described as a stress hormone, cortisol has other functions in macronutrient metabolism but can wreak havoc on body composition and muscle-building efforts by inducing muscle protein breakdown. Cortisol belongs to a larger family of hormones known as glucocorticoids, and high levels of these hormones may inhibit the action of the hormone leptin.[61] While cortisol is part of our daily diurnal rhythm or biological clock and we need some cortisol to function properly, too much cortisol can be detrimental to how we look and feel. When it comes to cortisol, we need a Goldilocks amount: not too much, not too little. Unfortunately, between our daily perceived stressors and the physical stress induced from dieting, cortisol often falls out of this healthy sweet spot.

Thyroid, leptin, insulin, ghrelin, testosterone, cortisol, and our entire endocrine system can be influenced in varying degrees by low-calorie dieting. Results from a number of studies indicate a general or expected hormonal response to restricted calorie intake, and a typical bodily response may include increased hunger and decreased metabolic rate while threatening existing levels of muscle mass. This is explained by reported decreases in leptin and insulin with lower body fat levels, compromised thyroid and testosterone levels, and increased ghrelin and cortisol. Simply put, calorie restriction is a recipe for more hunger, more stress, and less muscle.[62] No wonder dieting is difficult! Unfavorable changes in circulating hormone levels may even persist as subjects attempt to maintain a reduced body weight after the cessation of active weight loss.[63]

In the case of all the above hormones, the pattern is that each adapts to a perceived indication of lower energy availability and increased stress. The body is merely engaging in self-regulating processes to maintain stability by making metabolic and hormonal adjustments that are best for its survival in the current environmental conditions (food quantity, stress, threats, etc.). While it's clear that an attempt to restrict calories and reduce body fat causes a distinct hormonal environment, more research is needed to determine the chronic impact of these alterations in anabolic and catabolic hormones. These transient metabolic and hormonal changes appear to make weight maintenance more challenging, as well as promote weight regain and threaten lean mass retention. This throws a massive wrench in our attempts to maximize our body transformation efforts. To maximize diet success, we must manage these hormones to mitigate the unfavorable changes.

ADAPTATIONS TO ENERGY EXPENDITURE AND CALORIE OUTPUT

In earlier sections, we defined total daily energy expenditure (TDEE) as the combination of the calorie output from our resting metabolism (BMR/RMR) with additional energy burn or utilization coming from exercise activity (EAT), non-exercise activity or movement (NEAT), and the calories expended during the consumption, digestion, and assimilation of food (TEF). In response to weight loss, we see reductions in TDEE, BMR, EAT, NEAT, and TEF, but the reductions exceed the changes predicted by a drop in body weight. The aforementioned hormonal and metabolic changes could be the culprit. Previous research by Dr. Eric Trexler refers to this excessive drop in TDEE as adaptive thermogenesis. His research suggests that adaptive thermogenesis may promote the restoration of baseline body weight, which could help to explain the increasing difficulty experienced when weight loss plateaus despite low caloric intake and the propensity to regain weight after weight loss.[64]

Exercise activity thermogenesis also drops in response to weight loss. When it comes to any type of movement, we are using energy to move our body mass through space. A reduction in body mass will reduce the energy needed to complete a specific movement, exercise, or activity. Even when external weight is added to match baseline, pre-diet scale weight, energy expenditure to complete a given workload or activity remains below baseline. Even adding weight back "artificially" isn't enough to match prior energy expenditure. It has been speculated that this increase in this efficiency may be related to the hormonal and metabolic changes that accompany weight loss.

In the case of the calories burned in digestion and assimilation, the decreases in the thermic effect of food seem most straightforward and logical. Simply put, when we eat less food, we burn fewer calories digesting, assimilating, and absorbing food. Roughly 10% of energy expenditure is attributed to TEF, with values varying based on the macronutrient composition of the diet. While the relative magnitude of TEF does not appear to change with energy restriction, such dietary restriction involves the consumption of fewer total calories and therefore decreases the absolute magnitude of TEF.

Unlike the less drastic changes in thermic effect of food, non-exercise activity is more significantly affected by calorie restriction. NEAT also decreases with an energy deficit. Evidence suggests that spontaneous physical activity, a component of NEAT, is decreased in energy-restricted subjects and may remain suppressed for some time after subjects return to normal feeding. This basically means that the deeper you get into an energy deficit, the more you will be inclined to take the elevator instead of the stairs. You might blink, tap, or fidget less. This general decrease in your desire to move during the day is primarily a means of energy conservation. While it may seem like just a few motions and movements here or there, these small changes add up. Persistent suppression of NEAT may contribute to weight regain in the post-diet period.

These changes serve to minimize the energy deficit, attenuate further loss of body mass, and promote weight regain in weight-reduced subjects.[65] We cannot diet forever. But if we still have fat to lose, we need to look to tools like nutritional periodization and nonlinear dieting to unlock lasting success.

ADDRESSING ADAPTATION WITH NUTRITIONAL PERIODIZATION

Common practice in the diet industry is simply to subtract calories, move more, and repeat ad nauseum until desired results are achieved. For beginners who have a propensity toward overeating and inactivity, this practice is decent starting advice, but diet culture is not limited to this scenario. It could also be argued that even for those who are overweight, a slower approach might make things more sustainable and potentially avoid some of the ramifications outlined by the "Biggest Loser" study and the dietary rebound effect explained in the introductory chapters. On the other hand, for frequent dieters or seasoned veterans of diet culture, the metabolic adaptations outlined in the previous section make results harder to come by, even if these clients are not obese or severely overweight. This is a drawback of a linear dieting approach, where there's no break or strategic intervention to mitigate adaptation and maximize continued energy expenditure. This is where we can observe the power of nonlinear dieting in physique transformation and fat-loss efforts.

While nonlinear dieting has been practiced by athletes and bodybuilders for decades in different formats, this concept is novel for the general population of lifestyle dieters. Nonlinear dieting is also known as a form of intermittent *energy* restriction, which means we are not always trying to eat less than our body needs to maintain its weight. This strategy can be used to limit or thwart the adaptations seen with conventional diet models and thereby increase weight loss during subsequent periods of energy restriction.[66] Nonlinear dieting involves intermittent periods of energy balance throughout the diet as opposed to continuous long-term energy restriction. Non-linear dieting is an integral part of nutritional periodization or planning.

This strategy can be incorporated in various strategies of cycling caloric intake over daily or weekly time periods. While "adding food" seems like a simple concept, it is best accomplished through planned, healthy refeeding that takes into account an individual's psychological state and relationship with food. Think of this as an opportunity to eat slightly more calories and moderately increase portion size with nutrient-dense choices. It is not a dietary free-for-all or the appropriate time for you to challenge Takeru Kobayashi or Joey Chestnut to a hot dog-eating contest at Coney Island in New York City.

Examples of nonlinear dieting strategies include calorie or carbohydrate cycling, interval dieting, and planned diet breaks. Each strategy is slightly different in how it attempts to create a calorie deficit and then interrupt that hypocaloric state with higher quantities of energy, but protein intake often remains the same regardless, with the primary changes being made to carbohydrates or dietary fat. Calorie cycling accomplishes this by toggling daily intake across the week (for example, five days of a base intake and two days of slightly higher intake), whereas an interval diet toggles weekly or monthly intakes. For example, you might eat fewer calories for one or two weeks, followed by a maintenance phase for one to two weeks. An approach with a planned diet break might be six, eight, or twelve weeks of linear dieting in a hypocaloric state, followed by one or two weeks of an intake closer to maintenance calories.

One of the most frequently cited examples of nonlinear dieting methods is the MATADOR study. In this particular study, researchers examined a "two week on, two week off" approach to calorie restriction. This approach was later reviewed by researchers in 2019, where they maintained the consensus that avoiding extreme prolonged deficits and using nonlinear dieting with resistance training and a high protein intake is the best approach. While the 2018 and 2019 research focused largely on weekly adjustments in calorie intake, recent studies have studied the effects of intermittent energy restriction or nonlinear dieting when calorie intake is manipulated over a seven-day period split between five days of calorie restriction and two days of maintenance calorie consumption.[67] From anecdotal coaching experience as well as the strength of the data presented in this study, it seems most could benefit from the 5/2 level approach, and the process may feel less drawn out for the dieter than taking the MATADOR 2/2 approach. It is also worth noting that researchers have had a difficult time replicating the results of the original MATADOR study.

Readers should use these styles as potential tools for transformation progress rather than pledging unwavering allegiance to a particular method. The section below expands on nonlinear dieting practice examples.

EXAMPLES OF NONLINEAR DIETING OR NUTRITIONAL PERIODIZATION
CARBOHYDRATE OR CALORIE CYCLING

This approach adjusts energy intake on a daily basis by toggling the total amount of carbohydrates or calories consumed on specific days. Carb or calorie cycling can be accomplished with two or three different intakes. The amount of weekly calories consumed still matters here because cycling intake will not override total energy (calories) consumed across the week. It is a way to potentially emphasize certain training days, or accommodate social events or a varied lifestyle.

Monday	Tuesday	Wednesday	Thursday	Friday	Saturday	Sunday
Intake A	Intake B	Intake C	Intake A	Intake B	Intake C	Repeat

5/2 EATING

In this example, the two maintenance calorie days (intake Y) are placed on Friday and Saturday, whereas the lower calorie intake days are placed on Sunday through Thursday. The days of the week are adjustable, meaning any five days can be the lower intake, and any two days can be the higher intake. Once again, this approach is designed to mitigate metabolic adaptation and preserve lean muscle mass. It is not a magic trick and will still require adherence and effort.

Monday	Tuesday	Wednesday	Thursday	Friday	Saturday	Sunday
Intake X	Intake X	Intake X	Intake X	Intake Y	Intake Y	Intake X

INTERVAL DIETING/MATADOR

In weeks 1 and 2, intake X is a 20–30% reduction from the calories consumed to maintain your current body weight as assessed by a seven-day food journal.

Monday	Tuesday	Wednesday	Thursday	Friday	Saturday	Sunday
Intake X	Intake X	Intake X	Intake X	Intake X	Intake X	Intake X

In weeks 3 and 4, intake Y is maintenance calorie intake or, in other words, the intake level where you maintain your weight over a seven-day period (you'd need to track this maintenance level *prior* to starting an interval dieting approach).

Monday	Tuesday	Wednesday	Thursday	Friday	Saturday	Sunday
Intake Y	Intake Y	Intake Y	Intake Y	Intake Y	Intake Y	Intake Y

DIET BREAKS SPRINKLED THROUGHOUT LONGER DIET PHASES

In this example, you follow your diet as planned until progress stalls. For some, this might be six to eight weeks and include a week of maintenance calories when progress begins to stall or adherence becomes increasingly difficult. Some dieters may notice they can extend the diet longer, whereas others may need breaks every four or five weeks depending on their lifestyle and training practices. During this process, having a coach can be especially helpful because a coach will monitor biofeedback and training performance and gauge the appropriate time for this type of intervention.

USING BUILD, BURN, AND BREAK SEASONS OF NUTRITION METHODOLOGY

PLANNED DIET PHASES OR COMPETITION PHASES

An example of this is the twelve-to-sixteen-week diet phase using the nonlinear 5/2 method that was originally studied by Dr. Bill Campbell at the University of South Florida. The diet phase can end when either you have achieved your target level of fat loss or you can't get results on a 15% drop in carbs and fats and a 10–20% increase in activity (they use cardiovascular activity as their metric).[68] If results can't be achieved with these drops, this is likely a good indicator that your body isn't in the best place to continue dieting, and you should consider taking time to reverse diet to build up your metabolic rate.[69]

REVERSE OR RECOVERY DIET PHASES

During this phase, you gradually increase calories to a new

estimated maintenance. If quality of life and biofeedback have significantly deteriorated, a recovery diet might be the wise move, especially for individuals dieting without special assistance in the form of bioidentical hormone replacement (pharmaceutical interventions) or performance-enhancing drugs. For those who have dieted to a very low body fat percentage (think unsustainably lean photoshoot, competition, or meet prep), it may be necessary to regain 5–10% of your lowest weight within about eight weeks of the conclusion of your diet.

If you have intensely dieted to unsustainably low levels of body fat, then gaining some body fat may help to regain hormonal function. The difference between a reverse diet and a recovery diet is that the unsustainably lean individual needs to gain some weight and body fat using a recovery diet to alleviate symptoms of metabolic adaptation and the deteriorating quality of life that comes with severe calorie restriction. To regain weight more quickly, individuals may need to begin with their current maintenance calories plus 20–30%, with weekly or biweekly additions of 100–200 calories to keep the rate of gain trending in the direction of regaining 5–10% of the lowest weight achieved dieting.

Individuals who are not preparing for a competition or photoshoot and have not reached an unsustainably low body fat may prefer to raise their calories gradually to make future dieting attempts easier and to potentially elevate their maintenance calorie intake level over time. The allure of reverse dieting is that in many cases, when a gradual buildup of calories is achieved in an incremental fashion, dieters can ward off excess fat gain and dissipate some of the added calories through adaptive thermogenesis and NEAT. The same "metabolic adaptations" that work against us when subtracting calories can sometimes play to a dieter's advantage if they remain active and continue resistance training as calories are added in the reverse diet. This does not mean you can add food forever and not gain fat. It simply means that after the diet phase ends, a reverse diet can focus on ramping calories without sabotaging body composition.

When done correctly, reverse dieting affords a handful of metabolic benefits: BMR can climb, resulting in more energy expended. The ability to perform in workouts and exercise activity increases as a byproduct of consuming more calories (energy availability), and non-exercise activity often increases both subconsciously and consciously, resulting in the expenditure of more calories from movement outside of the gym or training sessions. In one study of lean individuals, eating 20% above maintenance calories did not significantly increase fat gain (whereas eating 40–60% above maintenance did).[70]

Best Practices for Reverse Dieting

Begin at current maintenance calories as a minimum (not predicted maintenance because this will be significantly skewed by your past diet efforts). If you have a healthy relationship with food and the scale and can handle changes in body composition, this intake could rise to 10–20% above where you are currently maintaining your weight to start.

If protein is adequate, begin replacing carbohydrates and fats evenly or in a percentage distribution based on personal preference. Most individuals will fall into a range of adding 50–150 calories to their daily intake on a weekly basis. Very petite individuals with lower dietary intakes may need to titrate this or make additions on a biweekly basis if looking to avoid more rapid fat accrual. Very large individuals with a lot of body mass may need to add higher amounts of carbohydrates or fat and closer to 200 calories or above. This can vary person to person, so take a week-by-week approach and audit your response to the incremental jumps in food intake.

For individuals participating in strength sports, sprinting, or high-intensity exercise or those looking to follow the research by the book, it might be beneficial to add calories from carbohydrates given low rates of fat turnover in fat cells after intense dieting or calorie restriction and preferential oxidation of carbohydrates during this time period. Essentially, adding calories with a slight tilt in favor of carbohydrates might reduce fat gain versus adding calories primarily from fat. While science is cool, remember personal preference and adherence is paramount, so if adding more carbohydrates isn't working for you, it is okay to adjust the approach to include more fat.

PLANNED MAINTENANCE PHASES

There will be seasons of life where dieting is not the number-one priority. Examples of this include seasons where stress might be higher or scheduling deviations and travel are more frequent. Other scenarios might include having a new child, getting a promotion at work, or a time period focused on family caregiving. The quantity of calories and food consumed during this phase should be an amount where, over the course of a seven-day food log and tracking scale weight, you maintain your weight. This is also a phase that can be used to emphasize training performance as the body will have more nutrients available than in a diet phase or season of calorie reduction.

PLANNED SURPLUS OR LEAN MUSCLE ACCRUAL PHASES

Some individuals will have times when they are looking to gain weight or increase the amount of muscle on their body. This is an example of a planned calorie surplus or improvement phase. The idea behind this season is to provide the body with more raw materials. If you wanted to build a bigger house, you would need more construction materials. To build a bigger, more muscular body, you need more nutrients.

Remember that without seasonal nutritional periodization, the body is primed to downregulate metabolic rate, and it subsequently becomes easier to store more body fat with the decreases observed in NEAT, EAT, and TEF. Becoming lean and staying lean without nutritional periodization requires a brute force and stringent approach that places additional focus and strain on the individual because of restricted food intake. Dieters who adhere to significant deficits may have constrained eating patterns as fewer deviations become feasible, and the maintenance calorie intake window will slowly shrink in metabolically adapted individuals over time. It may only be by a handful of calories, but without a reverse diet or a return to maintenance, these individuals are likely to face compounding issues with fatigue, energy levels, and more significant downregulation of their reproductive hormone axis and thyroid axis. Once these downregulations or adaptations have taken hold, a reverse diet followed by a maintenance period is necessary.

MAXIMIZE ADHERENCE

One of the final tools for managing your appetite and food decisions might surprise you. While Granny might have raised little Timmy on chicken nuggets and an absence of vegetables, this doesn't need to hold him back from his weight-loss pursuits. In fact, in a recent study, researchers discovered that cravings for high-calorie foods decreased during phases of weight loss and weight management. Engineering the right environment and creating traction in your transformation can not only propel you to some short-term results, but it can also lead to long-term changes in your preferences. Aside from maintaining an open mind to the changes in your palate, another key for sustainable success is flexibility within the diet.

In recent years, concepts like IIFYM (if it fits your macros) or "flexible dieting" have made significant headway. The idea behind these eating plans is if you eat the right amounts of macros and calories, you can substitute a variety of food choices to achieve your desired physical goals (note: I'm not encouraging the abandonment of micronutrient-dense food choices). Say you need to eat thirty grams of carbohydrates in a meal.

A flexible dieting approach means being able to substitute carbohydrate-equivalent foods or adjusting serving sizes of carbohydrate-containing foods to achieve that nutrient total. For example, I might choose from fruit, sweet potatoes, squash, rice, or another food to hit that particular macronutrient. Some follow this approach while incorporating nutrient-dense foods, while others fit treats and highly processed unconventional "diet foods" into their eating regimen.

Recent dietary restraint and self-regulation research discovered that dieters responded favorably to flexibility.[71] In fact, the less absolute or rigid the dieting rules (what some psychology professionals would refer to as an "all or nothing" mindset), the less likely participants were to fall off the wagon. Another study over a twenty-week period conducted by Laurin Conlin also showed that a flexible strategy is equally effective for weight loss during a calorie restricted diet in free-living, resistance-trained individuals.[72] It is worth noting that many of these studies comparing flexible vs. rigid eating styles will always be shorter than the many decades you will be consuming food during your lifetime. The important information to extract is that we can use a blended approach to avoid falling off the wagon and reverting to the yo-yo diet scenarios mentioned earlier in this book.

For the best possible results, flexibility in food choice should still incorporate nutrient-dense foods because hyperpalatable high-calorie meals with minimal nutrient density (think State Fair food, drive-throughs, or cafeteria concoctions) can potentially compromise four of the key principles in this book: managing appetite, maximizing absorption, minding micronutrients, and maximizing adherence (primarily because they can skyrocket cravings and make it more difficult to manage calorie intake). Hyperpalatable, low nutrient density foods might also be less optimal for cardiometabolic health and longevity if they are void of omega-3 fatty acids and essential vitamins and minerals. Think of flexibility as more of an opportunity to rotate and incorporate a variety of food choices that contain key nutrients like protein, vitamins, minerals, fats, and carbohydrates, as opposed to being viewed as a mechanism for sneaking seventeen different snacks into your daily diet in place of consuming a nutrient-dense plate at each meal. Flexibility also affords dieters the opportunity to have freedom to rotate foods as opposed to a singular redundant meal plan each day.

While this book outlines a number of strategies for important considerations like appetite, adherence, and absorption, be mindful that biting off more than you can chew (literally) will often lead to a dieter's demise. Rather than trying to incorporate every strategy from this book at once, implement one strategy at a time until it becomes a repeatable skill. For example, you might start by focusing on managing appetite with proper protein intake and attentive eating practices prior to practicing the incorporation of the other Ms.

MAXIMIZE ABSORPTION AND ASSIMILATION

Unlike their calorie-counting counterparts, the health and fitness industry is also filled with kombucha-drinking, fermented food fiends who would promise you that probiotics or a meticulous focus on your microbiome is the secret to a fit figure, a flat stomach, or more muscle. While it is true that each individual's microbiome is unique and that the gut is rather important, probiotics alone will certainly not bring you the lasting results you desire if you are not consciously engaging in other health-oriented behaviors like exercise and managing your nutrition (be mindful that these behaviors influence the gut as well). But paying attention to gut health and maximizing absorption of the food we eat is one surefire way to create additional leverage in your transformation and longevity pursuits.

Two thousand years ago, Hippocrates, who is often called *the father of medicine*, said that "bad digestion is at the root of all evil" and "death sits in the bowels." He continuously told the public and his followers that "all disease begins in the gut."

This man was clearly ahead of his time, and the microbiome is arguably a cornerstone of your metabolism and health of the entire human organism. Earlier in this book, we discussed how key nutrients and activities like walking can promote digestive health, but there's more to the story.

With millions of individuals suffering from irritable bowel disease[73] and millions more having regular digestive complaints such as acid reflux, bloating, gas, or discomfort, it is clear that digestive health is paramount. In the United States alone, sixty to seventy million people are affected by a digestive disease. The net impact of this economically results in the United States spending $141.8 billion a year dealing with all the digestive issues, and physicians alone wrote over 1.8 million pharmaceutical prescriptions to deal with those disorders. These issues are not solely limited to the United States, either. As of 2012, an estimated 10–20% of the UK population was or had been impacted by irritable bowel syndrome (IBS). A study published in the same year indicated that inflammatory bowel disease (IBD) is emerging as a global problem, with the incidence being far higher in Europe, North America, and other regions of the globe that have embraced the standard American diet (SAD).[74]

From a mechanical perspective, digestion begins in the mouth and ends near the colon, but there's more to the gut, digestion, and absorption than simply being a "pass-through entity" or "one-way street." Optimizing gastrointestinal health is essential in order to lower overall levels of inflammation in the body, improve the digestion of foods that we are eating so that we can properly absorb the nutrients from them, maximize the health of the immune system, and ensure our gut contains a healthy and balanced level of bacteria.

When it comes to optimizing digestion, not only our food choices but also activities like chewing, drinking appropriate amounts of water at the right times, and going for small post-meal walks can make a massive difference in how we look, feel, and assimilate our food. Gut complications can disrupt absorption of key vitamins and minerals essential to the function of our metabolism and the status of our hormones.

It is abundantly clear that gut health matters for how we feel and our nutrient status, but what about our looks? While this area needs continued exploration, initial research is powerful and promising. Studies at the Washington University School of Medicine in St. Louis on identical twins and mammals showed that by transplanting entire collections of human microbes into different groups of mice, the researchers could mimic the body composition of each twin.[75] Mice fed low-fat mouse chow and given gut microbes from an obese twin gained weight and fat and took on the metabolic dysfunction of the donor, while mice given gut microbes from a lean twin stayed lean. Throughout their experiments, the researchers found they could transmit an individual's body composition and associated metabolic dysfunction to the mice regardless of whether a donor's gut microbes were first grown in the laboratory or transferred from a fecal sample.[76] As with any other research, animal studies are more like tools for extrapolation and ideation for future research as opposed to providing the strength of evidence of a randomized human trial. So, before you go ask a fit friend for their gut microbes and to bring you a fresh stool sample, consider some of these basic steps to optimize gut health:

1. Deviate from the standard American diet, and choose micronutrient-dense whole foods.

2. Chew your food, and consider taking more time at each meal to eat attentively.

3. Consider implementing short post-meal walks (outside if possible).

4. Consider adjusting your meal spacing, and if you struggle with your blood glucose, consider taking twelve hours between your evening and morning meal or exploring time-restricted feeding if it works for you and improves cardiometabolic markers of health (like fasting insulin, A1C, triglycerides, etc.).

5. Adjust your fiber to individual adequacy and tolerance. This can range from 20–50 grams daily depending on your calorie intake. On average, research supports the inclusion of at least 14 grams per 1,000 calories for most individuals.

6. Diversify your food: eat a variety of colorful fruits and/or vegetables.

7. Incorporate fermented foods if you enjoy them.

8. Talk to your doctor about probiotic supplementation after any treatment that includes a course of prescription or intravenous antibiotics. A specific yeast-based probiotic called Saccharomyces can be beneficial when aggressive prescription antibiotic regimens or intravenous antibiotics are used.

MICRONUTRIENTS WITH MACRO-IMPORTANCE: MINDING MICRONUTRIENT STATUS

While you might think there's no common flaw between a ketogenic diet, a bodybuilder's diet, and a quick-fix cleanse approach to weight loss, one often-overlooked area plagues a multitude of eating styles across diet cultures: micronutrient deficiencies. Whether you are consuming a redundant repertoire of chicken, rice, and broccoli or living solely off beef, butter, and bacon, the inherent restriction and lack of variety leads to deficiencies in key vitamins and minerals. While you can certainly supplement to fill nutritional gaps, it is always advisable to make nutrient-dense food choices that are naturally packed with these vitamins and minerals.

COMMON DIETARY APPROACHES

NUTRIENTS TO CONSIDER

DIET	MAIN NUTRIENTS OF CONCERN		SOLUTION
GLUTEN FREE	Calcium Iron Magnesium Zinc	Folate Thiamin Vitamin B Vitamin B12	Include leafy greens, plenty of meats, eggs, nuts, yogurts, or cheeses
VEGAN	Calcium Iron	Zinc Vitamin B12	Include pumpkin seeds for zinc, bok choy for calcium, spinach for iron, and supplements for vitamin B12
KETO	Calcium Potassium Magnesium	Pantothenic Acid Copper Vitamin E	Include a large variety of meats, eggs, nuts and seeds, and leafy green vegetables
PALEO	Calcium Iodine	Riboflavin Thiamin	Include sardines (with bones for calcium), seaweed, bok choy, other leafy greens, and plenty of nuts and seeds
DAIRY FREE	Calcium		Include sardines with bones, bok choy, almonds, and other leafy greens
CARNIVORE	Vitamin C Vitamin A Vitamin E	Calcium Potassium Magnesium	Include a huge variety of ruminant, fowl, mollusks, shellfish, and eggs with a true nose-to-tail approach including all organs

We can see this nutritional deficiency in action in people on a plant-based diet, specifically veganism. Often plant-based eaters encounter a myriad of deficiencies, including vitamin D3, folate, zinc, iron, B12, and omega-3 essential fatty acids (EPA and DHA). A keto dieter might be missing out on folate, biotin, selenium, vitamin A, vitamin E, vitamin D, chromium, iodine, and magnesium. While there's plenty of middle ground between these two extremes, many dietary approaches will skew micronutrient status depending on the primary food groups consumed.

A great way to monitor your own micronutrient status is to use a tracking app like Cronometer. Another approach is to do a quick internet search for nutrition data for some of your favorite foods or meals to see what micronutrients you most commonly consume and where you might be lacking. Try not to get lost in the minutia of the microgram, but observe patterns and trends in eating behavior that may result in you missing out on key micronutrients.

While the prefix "micro" may make these nutrients seem less important, the truth is these vitamins and minerals are essential for day-to-day human function, from bolstering the immune system to serving as cofactors in reactions, strengthening bones and teeth, and healing wounds. You also rely on micronutrients to convert food to energy and repair cellular damage. You can work with your doctor or healthcare provider to test your micronutrient status periodically, as well as asking how certain health conditions, medications, and habits impact your levels. The elderly, pregnant women, athletes, and obese populations should all pay special attention to micronutrient deficiency risks.

In terms of testing, you can check the status of some micronutrients via regular blood work. For example, your doctor can order tests to check RBC magnesium levels and hydroxy vitamin D levels, as well as iron, ferritin, and total iron binding capacity (this is especially important if you are vegan or vegetarian). Once you have become aware of a potential deficiency risk or a tested deficiency for a particular micronutrient, you can take corrective action via dietary changes or strategic supplementation. For more on micronutrients, you can find the full "Micronutrient Mastery" series (aired from Summer–Fall 2021) on the podcast *Sam Miller Science* on Apple Podcasts and Spotify.

Potential micronutrient deficiencies certainly are not the only downfall of popular one-size-fits-all diet styles. In the next section, we will dive into the pros, cons, and pitfalls of popular diets and why they may or may not work for your particular situation or circumstances.

POPULAR DIETS: PROS, CONS, AND PITFALLS

This section includes many diet styles. Understand that a diet is simply a mechanism to manipulate total nutrition (caloric intake and macronutrient and micronutrient profile). Adequate nutrition can be achieved without any dietary label or fad. Dietary adherence is superior to dietary style in most cases. The emphasis here is that each form of nutritional manipulation has benefits and consequences. For example, if you were going to purchase a vehicle, both a convertible and an SUV have their unique benefits depending on your situation. Environment and context dictate everything. If you live in Southern California or Florida, you have more flexibility to choose the convertible. If you call Alaska or Canada home or have several children, you would benefit from the SUV. Do not look at dietary styles in a vacuum or silo. Consider the entire frame of exercise, lifestyle, and health history. With an intelligent strategy, nutrition can be manipulated in any form or fashion to achieve the same physical and physiological result as a fad diet with a prominent label.

TIME-RESTRICTED EATING OR INTERMITTENT FASTING

Pros: Fasting can lead to some insulin sensitivity improvements in insulin-resistant individuals, likely due to its ability to assist in creating a calorie deficit across the day or week and avoiding the constant stimulus of feeding. Some evidence shows that fasting may help with longevity or cellular cleanup processes known as autophagy, but gauging individual responses and assessing sustainability with this dietary protocol is essential. However, some of the autophagy-related benefits from fasting may stem from the fact that people who are fasting are often in a calorie deficit (which can also potentially push this same mechanism from a health perspective).

In terms of fat loss, for some individuals, fasting allows for better calorie compliance, consistency, and adherence over longer periods by requiring a commitment to a specific eating window. There is also evidence that implementing an eating window earlier in the day and stopping eating four to five hours before bed (e.g., 10:00 a.m. to 6:00 p.m.) may help regulate circadian rhythm and reduce markers of metabolic syndrome (insulin resistance) and cardiovascular disease in obese individuals, regardless of if weight is lost or not. The specific time window above is largely the brainchild of Satchin Panda, though many people have deviated from this particular window and still found success in their own health journey.

Cons: Fasting is typically not advised for people with hypothyroidism or serious adrenal issues. Be mindful that extended, repeated fasts signal the hypothalamus and pituitary that there is a lack of food. This typically is a bad idea for women who already have cycle irregularities or individuals under high stress.

If you have other medical conditions, have a chat with your doctor or find a specialist for your condition.

Anecdotally, men appear to respond differently to fasting than women; female physiology seems more sensitive to changes in energy as a hedge against the caloric cost of pregnancy and subsequent breastfeeding, though more research needs to be conducted to determine if this is true when examining broader segments of the population with varying levels of stress and exercise activity. Intermittent eating windows are also a poor choice for anyone with a history of an eating disorder or binge-eating tendencies because they can reinforce past behavior patterns of restrictive eating followed by a bolus of food.

THE KETOGENIC DIET

Pros: It may be helpful in managing epileptic seizures or creating a calorie deficit for individuals who achieve dietary adherence through a fat-rich dietary protocol or for individuals who face extreme lethargy or poor blood sugar control when consuming carbohydrates due to insulin resistance and are not willing to engage in intense exercise activity, or in situations where intense activity is contraindicated.

Cons: There appears to be a relationship between carbohydrate consumption, insulin, and the counter-regulatory nature of carbohydrate consumption with cortisol and the parasympathetic (rest and digest) nervous system. Keto does not support glycolytic activities or intense sports performance to the same degree that a carbohydrate-rich diet would. People often believe low-carb diets and keto are synonymous, but that is a misnomer. Many individuals do not follow a true ketogenic diet but rather a very low-carb diet or a high-protein/low-carb diet, which relies on gluconeogenesis—the conversion of protein to sugar—instead of primarily relying on dietary fat and ketones.

THE PALEO DIET

Pros: Minimally processed food may be helpful in reducing inflammatory reactions to dairy, gluten, or autoimmune triggers in cases such as Hashimoto's thyroiditis. Paleo choices are often nutrient-dense, which can be beneficial for individuals with micronutrient deficiencies or as a way to keep a list of food options short and simple. Some users forget that calories still must be equated to other diet options relative to an individual's TDEE (as explained in earlier sections).

Cons: Dietary adherence is more challenging for some. Many paleo zealots do not track macronutrients, making it harder to steer nutrition toward a calorie deficit or calorie surplus. Very active individuals who perform a high volume of intense training may need additional carbohydrate sources to replenish muscle glycogen (fuel storage) and optimize performance. This can be hard to do if you are eating only veggies, fruits, and some potatoes.

VEGANISM, VEGETARIANISM, OR PLANT-BASED EATING

Pros: For people who eat predominately vegetables, legumes, and fruits, this diet is rich in dietary fiber and polyphenols. Another pro is that there are vegan, vegetarian, or plant-based eaters who consume minimally processed, nutrient-dense foods.

Cons: Many vegan or vegetarian eaters fail to obtain adequate amounts of B vitamins, omega-3 fatty acids, iron, folate, essential amino acids, vitamin D, and other minerals like zinc and magnesium unless strategic supplementation is utilized. Even with a deliberate attempt to eat "healthy" and nutritious foods, vegans can face challenges in their nutrient status due to their diet being rich in compounds that inhibit absorption of nutrients (phytates).

In addition to the potential micronutrient deficiencies (even on a healthy version of the diet), a common issue is that many vegans or vegetarians are really more like "starchans," meaning that instead of opting for animal proteins, they choose carbohydrate-dense, processed foods that provide less key nutrients relative to the total amount of calories consumed. These foods are often highly palatable and can compromise calorie control (exhibit A: vegan nuggets, pasta, vegan chips, vegan cookies, etc.). It is also hard to consume enough high-quality protein for specific body composition goals, and many people require meticulous planning or heavy use of vegan protein powders.

MADE FOR MOVEMENT

With nutrition being the focal point of the first fourteen chapters of this book, it might seem like exercise has become the redheaded stepchild of transformations and metabolic health, but that couldn't be further from the truth. Movement as a whole, including exercise activity, can serve an important role in transformations far beyond the calories burned from exercise. All forms of movement, including exercise, can serve as levers to improve longevity, body composition, and mental and emotional health. Movement is also imperative for weight maintenance after a diet or fat-loss phase because it can help cement the results you have worked so hard to achieve.

When it comes to weight loss and health, many people associate this combination with cardiovascular exercise and dieting. This is in large part due to the volume of studies and research on cardiovascular exercise in prior decades, as well as the social stigma or stereotypes associated with lifting weights. People often view cardio as "heart healthy" and feel instant gratification when they see the "calorie burn" number go up on their machine of choice.

In recent decades, exercise has evolved from the basics of walking, swimming, running, biking, and lifting weights to include every flavor of fitness and infomercial "get fit" gadget you could possibly dream of. With so many options available, you can easily succumb to overwhelm and decision fatigue in deciding what is best for your goals.

Two very simple forms of movement promise profound benefits: walking and resistance training. This is not to say that you can never ride like a bat out of hell in a Soul Cycle spin class, cultivate your inner yogi, or master the breaststroke in the pool like Michael Phelps. In fact, you might very well enjoy these activities from time to time. However, if your goal is to look better, feel better, and move better, it is hard to beat the combination of walking and resistance training as the foundation of your movement pyramid. Feel free to add other fitness flavors as the icing on this cake, so long as it doesn't detract from your daily energy levels or recovery. For now, we will start by explaining the benefits of these two pillars of movement and how they positively impact your metabolism.

PILLAR 1: RESISTANCE TRAINING

Resistance training is typically any external resistance applied while exercising. In an ideal scenario, these are exercises that can be progressively overloaded as you perform the movements over time. This can be done with dumbbells, barbells, machines, kettlebells, cables, bands, or, in some cases, even basic bodyweight exercises. While resistance training inherently involves moving your body through space, what is special about it is that we not only reap the benefits of the calories burned during the exercise activity (EAT), but it primes our bodies to respond more favorably to future meals while packing a massive punch for our overall health. Don't worry; you won't need to lift like, or look like, seven-time Mr. Olympia, Arnold "The Terminator" Schwarzenegger to get the benefits of resistance training for your metabolism and overall health.

OVERALL HEALTH

Few activities can improve overall health markers and resilience like resistance training. From the young and healthy to the elderly, resistance training has profound effects on health markers and overall metabolism. Some researchers have gone as far as to consider resistance training as a form of medicine.

Skeletal muscle, which represents about 40% of body weight, influences a variety of metabolic risk factors, including obesity, dyslipidemia, type 2 diabetes, and cardiovascular disease.[77] Furthermore, muscle tissue is the primary site for glucose disposal—so much so that muscle loss specifically increases the risk of insulin resistance and related health issues. Not only does resistance training shine on its own, but it also seems to excel over other forms of training modalities.

In comparative studies, individuals participating in resistance training over a sixteen-week period lowered metabolic and cardiovascular markers more than flexibility training (a yoga-like regimen). The resistance training groups experienced improvements in HDL and LDL (markers for cholesterol) and fasting insulin (a marker of metabolic syndrome and diabetes).[78] Additionally, when compared to walking, biking, or running, resistance training had better outcomes. While both activities reduced cardiovascular disease risk by 30–70%, the associations were strongest in the resistance training group.

QUALITY OF LIFE AND ANTI-AGING

After six months of resistance training, older adult participants (mean age of sixty-eight years) experienced gene expression reversal that resulted in mitochondrial characteristics similar to those in moderately active young adults (mean age of twenty-four years). The favorable changes observed in 179 genes associated with age and exercise led the researchers to conclude that resistance training can reverse aging factors in skeletal muscle.[79]

PHYSICAL DEVELOPMENT AND FRAILTY

Muscle can also serve as a potential predictor for longevity. *The American Journal of Medicine* and a significant volume of scholarly literature has examined the relationship between skeletal muscle and considerations such as healthspan or lifespan. From a common sense perspective, it seems logical that being able to withstand falls or having substantial strength relative to body weight could be especially beneficial in elderly individuals. Dr. Peter Attia utilizes measures of grip strength and eccentric strength to assess health and longevity, which makes a lot of sense when you consider a scenario such as an elderly man descending stairs and needing to control his weight or grab and hold a banister to prevent a nasty fall. One wrong move, and this scenario could result in hospitalization and exposure to sick individuals, bringing on an onslaught of complications. As an individual with parents in their seventies and eighties,

I've seen this play out firsthand, so I can't overstate the benefits of building muscle for both resilience and quality of life throughout the lifespan.

MUSCLE AS AN ENDOCRINE ORGAN

Many of the cardiometabolic benefits explained above can be attributed to muscle having "endocrine" or hormone-like effects across the body in terms of signaling and communicating with other glands and tissues. When you contract skeletal muscle, it releases myokines, or compounds that slow skin aging and improve carbohydrate metabolism, brain neurogenesis, fat metabolism, immune system function, and bone mass. While looking good in a swimsuit or boardshorts may be a goal of yours, it is only a secondary outcome to a much more important function of muscle as an organ of longevity. Remember, two key aspects of building skeletal muscle are resistance training and eating a protein-rich diet. While resistance training can come in different shapes and sizes, it is important to train intensely and challenge yourself to release these beneficial myokines mentioned earlier. To maximize recovery from this training, protein should be high quality, meaning it contains all nine essential amino acids. This type of protein can be found in animal foods, whey protein, vegan proteins made of pea and rice, and animal by-products such as dairy and eggs.

PILLAR 2: WALKING

Possibly the most accessible, feasible, and affordable type of movement for the vast majority of individuals is walking. Despite the lack of curb appeal, walking packs a powerful punch when added to your health and fitness regimen. This is largely due to the fact that it ramps up your NEAT. It makes sense that movement of any kind requires energy and therefore burns calories, but what evidence do we have to show that walking is beneficial for our health and body composition efforts?

Something as simple as interrupting prolonged sitting with brief bouts of light walking attenuates post-meal glucose responses, insulin levels, and triglycerides in type 2 diabetes patients. Fifty to seventy minutes of walking three days per week lowered visceral fat, abdominal fat, and improved glucose levels and inflammatory markers.[80] In fact, regular activity (not just exercise or resistance training) has such a potent effect on health it has suggested use as an alternative or adjunct to prescription drug therapy. Across forty-two studies involving 1843 participants who engaged in regular walking, researchers found that walking can lead to positive changes in resting heart rate, body fat, total cholesterol, depression, and quality of life for physical functioning.

In addition to the physical and metabolic changes illustrated above, walking can be a great tool for promoting digestion and alleviating the dreaded post-meal bloat or gastrointestinal discomfort. With over sixty-two million individuals in the United States struggling with digestive disease (going far beyond mild discomfort), something as simple as walking can be a fantastic intervention for health. Plus, I'm sure we can all remember a time when we've had a bit of a "food baby" or distended stomach from overindulgence or taking Thanksgiving a bit too far.

In a 2021 controlled trial, ninety-four participants were either given prokinetic medication or walked ten to fifteen minutes after a meal.[81] During this four-week study, both walking and medication resulted in significant improvements in GI tract symptoms such as belching, bloating, gas, and abdominal discomfort. When it came to post-meal fullness and bloating, walking was superior to prokinetic medication. With the significant spend on gut issues and GI medications, like proton pump inhibitors and acid reflux medication, it might be worth taking a stroll after that large meal to improve gut symptoms. Not to mention that getting your steps in boasts significant benefits for your sanity and body composition!

CREATING A RECIPE
FOR SUCCESS

With divergent opinions in diet culture, creating a game plan for success can be tiresome, frustrating, and filled with uncertainty—to the point where even creating this book and dissecting various approaches and viewpoints was no small task. It is important to remember that generalized advice can only take you so far, and there's no replacement for having a coach custom tailor a protocol to your individual health history, but I designed this section to give you some example strategies for getting started, no matter your background or situation. This section was incredibly hard to refine and share openly as a static content piece in a book for the masses. As an author who was a coach first, I understand that designing a successful program is highly dynamic and dependent on the context of your life, your health history, and your ability to adhere to the program recommendations.

Any of the suggested approaches can be used to build muscle or lose body fat. Think of them as scalable baseline recommendations that can be refined over time. To create a baseline awareness of current intake, keep a handwritten or digital food journal or food log for three to seven days using an app like MyFitnessPal, Macros+, or Cronometer. Cronometer offers the perk of micronutrient insights, which can be valuable for looking at multiple dimensions of nutrition beyond calorie consumption. Beginners may find more traction with a basic list or note of meals eaten, whereas intermediate to advanced dieters would derive the most benefit from diligent tracking and using the aforementioned technology.

All three ability levels outlined below should include the seasons of nutrition in their approach. The pillar components of the protocol focus less on individual calorie targets and more on keystone activities for sustainable health and body composition improvements. However, tracking your food for the suggested time period outlined above will give you insights into food consumption and where you land from a calorie and macronutrient intake perspective. Many of these foundational habits will help you achieve more sustainable success or have an easier time entering a calorie deficit if fat loss is your primary goal.

THE GREENHORN

- Walk five or more days per week for a minimum of twenty to thirty minutes. Walking is a very accommodating and scalable form of exercise for all populations. Consider taking your phone calls outside, listening to books or music, or simply enjoying a nature walk. An option to track your progress here would be to begin tracking your steps.
- Consider placing one short walk in the morning to maximize morning sun exposure when possible and one after

large meals, ideally outside when sunlight is present. If you struggle with precise timing, focus less on when the walk is and walk when it is most convenient for you.

- Eat protein at each meal, and aim to consume a minimum of three to four palm-sized portions of protein daily.
- Begin implementing good sleep hygiene practices: slowly back away from technology no less than thirty minutes to an hour prior to bedtime. Keep your sleeping area cool and dark. Leave ample time for shut-eye and shoot for more than seven hours.
- Begin resistance training two days per week. This can include beginner-friendly options like bodyweight workouts or bands. If this is your first time getting active, start with the walks and scale up to the resistance training over time as you begin moving more consistently with greater ease.
- If you are new to resistance training, consider grabbing a copy of *Science of Strength Training* by Austin Current or *The Resistance Training Revolution* by Sal Di Stefano to get started. Hire a coach or trainer for yourself if you need more support.
- Pay special attention to limiting distractions at meals so that you can eat attentively at a moderate pace. Consider pulling away from the television or parking your smartphone away from your plate.
- Pick one of these to start that you can confidently implement. Don't worry about perfecting all five to six practices at once.

THE INTERMEDIATE ENTHUSIAST

- Walking daily is the foundation of non-exercise movement. From a cumulative perspective, we are shooting for a daily non-exercise activity total of approximately eight thousand steps (ideally outside). This is not a "magic number" per se, but achieving an ample step count is cardioprotective and can help ward off just about any unfavorable health outcome ranging from depression to chronic disease. Consider including a short daily walk in morning sunlight as frequently as possible for physical, mental, and circadian health. If weight loss is your goal, you may need to add either longer or more frequent walks to increase your NEAT (defined earlier in the book) to raise energy expenditure.

- Implement resistance training three to four days per week. Consider using free weights, cables, machines, and body-weight exercises that allow for progression over time in weight lifted as well as total repetitions.

- Consume between 1g of protein per pound of lean body mass or up to 1g per pound of body weight (for those with a lot of weight to lose, lean body mass or goal body weight may be a more realistic target).

- Practice attentive eating by limiting distractions such as television and electronics. For an extra satiety boost we can add foods like fruits that you enjoy and/or vegetables that you can digest well, but protein intake and attentive eating are the essential foundations for most individuals.

- Participate in a deliberate weekly stress management activity: spend time in nature or with pets, meditate, or do creative therapy (art/music). Pick what resonates most with you and fits well in your life. If scheduling time to do it seems stressful, it probably means you need to pick a different stress management activity.

- Get a minimum of seven to eight hours of sleep per night, with similar wake and sleep times to maintain sleep hygiene and circadian rhythm.

- Add cardiovascular activity one to two times per week for

general health purposes, but do not view this as the primary tool for fat loss or physique changes.

- Begin using the seasons of nutrition to alternate time spent in dieting phases and recovery phases. Remember, the goal is to optimize your metabolic rate and metabolic health long-term rather than race to the lowest calorie intake possible.
- Optional but recommended: tracking macronutrients, fiber, water, and total calorie consumption.

THE ADVANCED ENTHUSIAST OR ATHLETE

- Walk seven days per week, somewhere in the neighborhood of eight thousand steps minimum, ideally performing a significant amount of this walking outdoors in the morning and early afternoon hours. This can be especially helpful if you are struggling to get on a consistent sleep schedule.
- Engage in resistance training four or five days per week; you may need to enlist the support of a coach to tailor programming to your specific needs or continue to reference the aforementioned books to implement a proper lifting program.
- Consume 1g of protein per pound of body weight. Note that individuals can go up to as high as 1.2–1.5g per pound during intense dieting phases to preserve muscle mass and help with appetite management.
- Nutritional periodization is a *must* for advanced athletes, dieters, and trainees. Focus on balancing your nutritional strategy across the year with ample time at your maintenance intake in addition to any time spent in a deficit or surplus. This means incorporating build, burn, and break phases. Even the most advanced athletes need breaks or deloads.
- Ramp dietary fiber as your digestive system allows. Research

supports the notion that consuming at least 14g per 1,000 calories is beneficial, but individual tolerance may vary. Some of the research-supported benefits of fiber may also be due to what is known as consuming a *whole food matrix* more than fiber intake on its own. For example, blueberries and other fruits contain fiber, but fruit is micronutrient and antioxidant dense as well, which contributes to overall health and well-being.

- Consider emphasizing carbohydrates and protein in the pre- and post-workout window to maximize nutrient uptake and boost training performance. In practice, this might be a carbohydrate and protein snack or meal surrounding your most strenuous workouts. Be mindful of the fact that high fats and fiber might not digest as well or serve to optimize performance in these pre- and post-workout settings.

- Participate in a deliberate weekly stress management activity: spend time in nature or with pets, meditate, journal, or do creative therapy (art/music). Pick what resonates most with you to manage stress and find joy. Typically the best activities will bring you out of rumination mode and back into the present moment and to be where your feet are.

- Get a minimum of eight hours of sleep per night, with similar wake and sleep times.

- Add cardiovascular exercise activity for general health purposes, but understand it is not the primary tool to focus on for body composition change.

- Progressing from intermediate to advanced may require strategic direction from a coach, or you may need to seek out more tools and knowledge beyond this book. My podcast (*Sam Miller Science*), social media (@sammillerscience), and website provide additional content that you can leverage for your goals.

In the three sample levels above, be mindful that each list is built off what is optimal for most people as indicated by nutrition and exercise research and exists on a gradient spectrum more so than three fixed ability levels. If you are trying to adopt any of these activities for the first time, prioritize a select few, and then gradually stack more health behaviors or activities on top of the ones you have already mastered. For example, let's say you love walks. That's great. Then maybe you move toward working on your sleep and wake times or eating an appropriate amount of protein for your goals. Already crushing the protein and water? Consider adding a stress management activity or some movement like walks or resistance training. While similar activities and choices drive results with your health and fitness, the order of operations will vary from person to person based on your existing lifestyle and health history. Consider enrolling an accountability partner or enlisting the support of a coach as you strive for more challenging goals that push you beyond your previous baseline behaviors.

There are circumstances where adjustments to these starting recommendations will be needed. For example, many female clients experiencing menopause or individuals who are insulin resistant see slightly better results with higher non-exercise activity goals like walking. The suggested activities in this book do not need to remain static, and can change over time based on your personal experience and implementation.

FINAL THOUGHTS

In a world of quick fixes and instant gratification, it is all too tempting to sign up for the latest health, fitness, or diet trend. In an industry that seems to thrive on overstated promises, the harsh reality is that many programs are not designed in alignment with our current knowledge and research on human metabolism or successful coaching practices. In fact, not only are many of these fad offerings not in alignment with the science of how our bodies work, but often these programs and protocols are in direct opposition to the constrained or compensatory nature of metabolism. While many people might glean short-lived results with some of the latest gimmicky, popularized approaches, we find true staying power when we harness our current understanding of the body's adaptive physiology to achieve our physical goals (weight loss, muscle gain, improved performance, etc.). This requires an understanding of and sensitivity to the nature of our body's interaction with two primary variables: stress and energy. In this book, you have learned information spanning from the origin of the calorie to the body's unique response to different food- and movement-related choices.

Discovering a nutrition and fitness approach that works for you should account for your life stress, your preferred training modalities, your digestive tolerance, and your current relationship with food and exercise. Regardless of everyone's unique preferences, a few common themes remain true. Nonlinear dieting featuring a focus on protein consumption paired with resistance training and non-exercise movement like walking seems to be our best recipe for success when it comes to fat loss, body recomposition, and muscle gain. This combination thwarts muscle loss, maximizes fat loss, and alleviates or mitigates many of the metabolic adaptations seen compared to individuals who are perpetually pursuing a calorie deficit to try to lose body fat. Energy management (a.k.a. calorie control) is critical, but dieters must understand that a controlled, planned calorie deficit for fat loss is vastly different from perpetual attempts at a calorie deficit. Calories, like many other units of measurement, require context. In order to yield our body's best possible response to dieting, we should spend time considering how to maximize adherence, manage appetite, mind micronutrients, mitigate adaptation, and maximize absorption of nutrients. We should not spend time perpetually dieting.

As mentioned in the introduction, the intention of this book was not to provide a cookie-cutter plan or to replace having a coach or professional lead you through this process. The goal was to create awareness and enhance your thought process for future decision-making. You now have a level of knowledge that allows for clarity and discernment in a world of fads, false promises, and questionable quick fixes. Perhaps in the past you were fooled, but now you are armed with the knowledge to spot red flags and overstated claims and help others do the same. You can continue to enhance your knowledge by accessing some of my other no-cost content like the four hundred-plus episodes of my podcast (*Sam Miller Science*), Instagram (@sammillerscience), or my personal website (www.sammillerscience.com). If you are a coach or health professional interested in learning from our more advanced content, visit www.metabolismschool.com.

Over the course of your lifetime, you will witness many diet trends come and go. The true test is not just reading this book and learning how to simplify metabolism. The true test is staying true to the simple path when you become inundated with marketing messages or gimmicks promising eight-minute abs, glorious glutes, and fret-free five-minute fat loss. Before embarking on any future fitness or nutrition quest, ask yourself if the program respects the pillars and principles you have learned in your journey to simplify health, fitness, nutrition, and metabolism.

If you have made it this far, thank you for reading *Metabolism Made Simple*.

The journey doesn't stop here! I've created more transformation tools and free resources to help you make sense of nutrition so that you can transform your metabolic health!

To download your free transformation tools and access resources, scan the code below, or visit www.metabolismmadesimple.com/more.

REFERENCES

Abraham, S. B., D. Rubino, N. Sinaii, S. Ramsey, and L. K. Nieman. "Cortisol, Obesity, and the Metabolic Syndrome: A Cross-Sectional Study of Obese Subjects and Review of the Literature." Obesity 21, no. 1 (January 2013): E105–E117. https://doi.org/10.1002/oby.20083.

Almstedt, Hawley C., Jacqueline A. Canepa, David A. Ramirez, and Todd C. Shoepe. "Changes in Bone Mineral Density in Response to 24 Weeks of Resistance Training in College-Age Men and Women." *Journal of Strength and Conditioning Research* 25, no. 4 (April 2011): 1098–103. https://doi.org/10.1519/jsc.0b013e3181d09e9d.

American College of Sports Medicine, Wojtek J. Chodzko-Zajko, David N. Proctor, Maria A. Fiatarone Singh, Christopher T. Minson, Claudio R. Nigg, George J. Salem, and James S. Skinner. "American College of Sports Medicine Position Stand. Exercise and Physical Activity for Older Adults." *Medicine & Science in Sports & Exercise* 41, no. 7 (July 2009): 1510–30. https://doi.org/10.1249/mss.0b013e3181a0c95c.

Aragon, Alan Albert and Brad Jon Schoenfeld. "Nutrient Timing Revisited: Is There a Post-Exercise Anabolic Window?" *Journal of the International Society of Sports Nutrition* 10, no. 1 (January 29, 2013): 5. https://doi.org/10.1186/1550-2783-10-5.

Arciero, Paul J., Michael J. Ormsbee, Christopher L. Gentile, Bradley C. Nindl, Jonathan R. Brestoff, and Maxwell Ruby. "Increased Protein Intake and Meal Frequency Reduces Abdominal Fat During Energy Balance and Energy Deficit." *Obesity (Silver Spring)* 21, no. 7 (July 2013): 1357–66. https://doi.org/10.1002/oby.20296.

Asgari Mehrabadi, Milad, Iman Azimi, Fatemeh Sarhaddi, Anna Axelin, Hannakaisa Niela-Vilén, Saana Myllyntausta, Sari Stenholm, Nikil Dutt, Pasi Liljeberg, and Amir M. Rahmani. "Sleep Tracking of a Commercially Available Smart Ring and Smartwatch Against Medical-Grade Actigraphy in Everyday Settings: Instrument Validation Study." *JMIR mHealth and uHealth* 8, no. 10 (November 2, 2020): e20465. https://pubmed.ncbi.nlm.nih.gov/33038869/.

Axelsson, John, Michael Ingre, Göran Kecklund, Mats Lekander, Kenneth P. Wright, and Tina Sundelin. "Sleep as Motivation: A Potential Mechanism for How Sleep Deprivation Affects Behavior." *Sleep* 43, no. 6 (June 15, 2020): zsz291. https://doi.org/10.1093/sleep/zsz291.

Ballor, D. L., V. L. Katch, M. D. Becque, and C. R. Marks. "Resistance Weight Training During Caloric Restriction Enhances Lean Body Weight Maintenance." *The American Journal of Clinical Nutrition* 47, no. 1 (January 1988): 19–25. https://doi.org/10.1093/ajcn/47.1.19.

Barry, Benjamin K. and Richard G. Carson. "The Consequences of Resistance Training for Movement Control in Older Adults." *The Journals of Gerontology: Series A, Biological Sciences and Medical Sciences* 59, no. 7 (July 2004): 730–54. https://doi.org/10.1093/gerona/59.7.m730.

Bianco, Antonio C., Domenico Salvatore, Balázs Gereben, Marla J. Berry, and P. Reed Larsen. "Biochemistry, Cellular and Molecular Biology, and Physiological Roles of the Iodothyronine Selenodeiodinases." *Endocrine Reviews* 23, no. 1 (February 2002): 38–89. https://doi.org/10.1210/edrv.23.1.0455.

Blair, Steven N. and Andrew S. Jackson. "Physical Fitness and Activity as Separate Heart Disease Risk Factors: A Meta-Analysis." *Medicine & Science in Sports & Exercise* 33, no. 5 (May 2001): 762–64. https://doi.org/10.1097/00005768-200105000-00013.

Boyle, James P., Theodore J. Thompson, Edward W. Gregg, Lawrence E. Barker, and David F. Williamson. "Projection of the Year 2050 Burden of Diabetes in the US Adult Population: Dynamic Modeling of Incidence, Mortality, and Prediabetes Prevalence." *Population Health Metrics* 8 (October 22, 2010). https://doi.org/10.1186/1478-7954-8-29.

Braun, Theodore P. and Daniel L. Marks. "The Regulation of Muscle Mass by Endogenous Glucocorticoids." *Frontier in Physiology* 6 (February 3, 2015): 12. https://doi.org/10.3389/fphys.2015.00012.

Broeder, C. E., K. A. Burrhus, L. S. Svanevik, and J. H. Wilmore. "The Effects of Either High-Intensity Resistance or Endurance Training on Resting Metabolic Rate." *The American Journal of Clinical Nutrition* 55, no. 4 (April 1992): 802–10. https://doi.org/10.1093/ajcn/55.4.802.

Bussau, Vanessa A., Timothy J. Fairchild, Arjun Rao, Peter Steele, and Paul A. Fournier. "Carbohydrate Loading in Human Muscle: An Improved 1 Day Protocol." *European Journal of Applied Physiology* 87, no. 3 (July 2002): 290–95. https://doi.org/10.1007/s00421-002-0621-5.

Buxton, Orfeu M., Milena Pavlova, Emily W. Reid, Wei Wang, Donald C. Simonson, and Gail K. Adler. "Sleep Restriction for 1 Week Reduces Insulin Sensitivity in Healthy Men." *Diabetes* 59, no. 9 (September 2010): 2126–33. https://doi.org/10.2337/db09-0699.

Bweir, Salameh, Muhammed Al-Jarrah, Abdul-Majeed Almalty, Mikhled Maayah, Irina V. Smirnova, Lesya Novikova, and Lisa Stehno-Bittel. "Resistance Exercise Training Lowers HbA1c More than Aerobic Training in Adults with Type 2 Diabetes." *Diabetology & Metabolic Syndrome* 1 (December 10, 2009): 27. https://doi.org/10.1186/1758-5996-1-27.

Byrne, N. M., A. Sainsbury, N. A. King, A. P. Hills, and R. E. Wood. "Intermittent Energy Restriction Improves Weight Loss Efficiency in Obese Men: The MATADOR Study." *International Journal of Obesity* 42 (August 17, 2017): 129–38. https://doi.org/10.1038/ijo.2017.206.

Campbell, Bill I., Danielle Aguilar, Lauren Colenso-Semple, Kevin Hartke, Chris Gai, David Gaviria, John Gorman, Josh Rubio, Adam Ibrahim, and Bobby Barker. "The Effects of Intermittent Carbohydrate Re-Feeds vs. Continuous Dieting on Body Composition in Resistance Trained Individuals: A Flexible Dieting Study." *Journal of the International Society of Sports Nutrition* 15 (November 6, 2018): 1–37. https://doi.org/10.1186/s12970-018-0256-5.

Campbell, W. W., M. C. Crim, V. R. Young, and W. J Evans. "Increased Energy Requirements and Changes in Body Composition with Resistance Training in Older Adults." *The American Journal of Clinical Nutrition* 60, no. 2 (August 1994): 167–75. https://doi.org/10.1093/ajcn/60.2.167.

Can, Yekta Said, Heather Iles-Smith, Niaz Chalabianloo, Deniz Ekiz, Javier Fernández-Álvarez, Claudia Repetto, Giuseppe Riva, and Cem Ersoy. "How to Relax in Stressful Situations: A Smart Stress Reduction System." *Healthcare* 8, no. 2 (April 16, 2020): 100. https://doi.org/10.3390/healthcare8020100.

Castaneda, Carmen, Jennifer E. Layne, Leda Munoz-Orians, Patricia L. Gordon, Joseph Walsmith, Mona Foldvari, Ronenn Roubenoff, Katherine L. Tucker, and Miriam E. Nelson. "A Randomized Controlled Trial of Resistance Exercise Training to Improve Glycemic Control in Older Adults with Type 2 Diabetes." *Diabetes Care* 25, no. 12 (December 2002): 2335–41. https://doi.org/10.2337/diacare.25.12.2335.

Cauza, Edmund, Ursula Hanusch-Enserer, Barbara Strasser, Bernhard Ludvik, Sylvia Metz-Schimmerl, Giovanni Pacini, Oswald Wagner, Petra Georg, Rudolf Prager, Karam Kostner, Attila Dunky, and Paul Haber. "The Relative Benefits of Endurance and Strength Training on the Metabolic Factors and Muscle Function of People with Type 2 Diabetes Mellitus." *Archives of Physical Medicine and Rehabilitation* 86, no. 8 (August 2005): 1527–33. https://doi.org/10.1016/j.apmr.2005.01.007.

Chinoy, Evan D., Joseph A. Cuellar, Kirbie E. Huwa, Jason T. Jameson, Catherine H. Watson, Sara C. Bessman, Dale A. Hirsch, Adam D. Cooper, Sean P. A. Drummond, and Rachel R. Markwald. "Performance of Seven Consumer Sleep-Tracking Devices Compared with Polysomnography." *Sleep* 44, no. 5 (May 14, 2021): zsaa291. https://doi.org/10.1093/sleep/zsaa291.

Coelho do Vale, Rita, Rik Pieters, and Marcel Zeelenberg. "The Benefits of Behaving Badly on Occasion: Successful Regulation by Planned Hedonic Deviations." *Journal of Consumer Psychology* 26, no. 1 (January 2016): 17–28. https://doi.org/10.1016/j.jcps.2015.05.001.

Conley, Michael S. and Michael H. Stone. "Carbohydrate Ingestion/ Supplementation or Resistance Exercise and Training." *Sports Medicine* 21, no. 1 (January 1996): 7–17. https://doi. org/10.2165/00007256-199621010-00002.

Cornelissen, Véronique A. and Robert H. Fagard. "Effect of Resistance Training on Resting Blood Pressure: A Meta-Analysis of Randomized Controlled Trials." *Journal of Hypertension* 23, no. 2 (February 2005): 251–59. https://doi.org/10.1097/00004872-200502000-00003.

Costamagna, Domiziana, Paola Costelli, Maurilio Sampaolesi, and Fabio Penna. "Role of Inflammation in Muscle Homeostasis and Myogenesis." *Mediators of Inflammation* 2015 (2015): 805172. https://doi. org/10.1155/2015/805172.

DiNicolantonio, James J. and James H. O'Keefe. "Importance of Maintaining a Low Omega-6/Omega-3 Ratio for Reducing Inflammation." *Open Heart* 5, no. 2 (November 26, 2018): e000946. https://doi.org/10.1136/openhrt-2018-000946.

DiNicolantonio, James J. and James H. O'Keefe. "Importance of Maintaining a Low Omega-6/Omega-3 Ratio for Reducing Platelet Aggregation, Coagulation and Thrombosis." *Open Heart* 6, no. 1 (May 2, 2019): e001011. https://doi.org/10.1136/openhrt-2019-001011.

DiNicolantonio, James J. and James H. O'Keefe. "The Importance of Maintaining a Low Omega-6/Omega-3 Ratio for Reducing the Risk of Autoimmune Diseases, Asthma, and Allergies." *Missouri Medicine* 118, no. 5 (September–October 2021): 453–59. https://pubmed.ncbi.nlm.nih. gov/34658440/.

DiNicolantonio, James J. and James H. O'Keefe. "Omega-6 Vegetable Oils as a Driver of Coronary Heart Disease: The Oxidized Linoleic Acid Hypothesis." *Open Heart* 5, no. 2 (September 26, 2018): e000898. https:// doi.org/10.1136/openhrt-2018-000898.

Doucet, Eric, Sylvie St-Pierre, Natalie Alméras, Jean-Pierre Després, Claude Bouchard, and Angelo Tremblay. "Evidence for the Existence of Adaptive Thermogenesis During Weight Loss." *British Journal of Nutrition* 85, no. 6 (June 2001): 715–23. https://doi.org/10.1079/bjn2001348.

Du, Chen, Megan Chong Hueh Zan, Min Jung Cho, Jenifer I. Fenton, Pao Ying Hsiao, Richard Hsia, Laura Keaver, Chang-Chi Lai, HeeSoon Lee, Mary-Jon Ludy, Wan Shen, Winnie Chee Siew Swee, Jyothi Thrivikraman, Kuo-Wei Tseng, Wei-Chin Tseng, Stephen Doak, Sara Yi Ling Folk, and Robin M. Tucker. "Evidence of Sleep Quality and Resilience on Perceived Stress, Dietary Behaviors, and Alcohol Misuse: A Mediation-Moderation Analysis of Higher Education Students from Asia, Europe, and North America during the COVID-19 Pandemic." *Nutrients* 13, no. 2 (January 29, 2021): 442. https://doi.org/10.3390/nu13020442.

Dunstan, David W., Robin M. Daly, Neville Owen, Damien Jolley, Maximilian De Courten, Jonathan Shaw, and Paul Zimmet. "High-Intensity Resistance Training Improves Glycemic Control in Older Patients with Type 2 Diabetes." *Diabetes Care* 25, no. 10 (October 2002): 1729–36. https://doi.org/10.2337/diacare.25.10.1729.

Edwards, Meghan K. and Paul D. Loprinzi. "Experimental Effects of Brief, Single Bouts of Walking and Meditation on Mood Profile in Young Adults." *Health Promotion Perspectives* 8, no. 3 (July 7, 2018): 171–78. https://doi.org/10.15171/hpp.2018.23.

Ewert, Alan and Yun Chang. "Levels of Nature and Stress Response." *Behavioral Sciences* 8, no. 5 (May 17, 2018): 49. https://doi.org/10.3390/bs8050049.

Farshchi, H. R., M. A. Taylor, and I. A. Macdonald. "Decreased Thermic Effect of Food After an Irregular Compared with a Regular Meal Pattern in Healthy Lean Women." *International Journal of Obesity and Related Metabolic Disorders* 28, no. 5 (May 2004): 653–60. https://doi.org/10.1038/sj.ijo.0802616.

Farshchi, H. R., M. A. Taylor, and I. A. Macdonald. "Regular Meal Frequency Creates More Appropriate Insulin Sensitivity and Lipid Profiles Compared with Irregular Meal Frequency in Healthy Lean Women." *European Journal of Clinical Nutrition* 58, no. 7 (July 2004): 1071–77. https://doi.org/10.1038/sj.ejcn.1601935.

Fastame, Maria Chiara, Marilena Ruiu, and Ilaria Mulas. "Hedonic and Eudaimonic Well-Being in Late Adulthood: Lessons from Sardinia's Blue Zone." *Journal of Happiness Studies* 23 (July 6, 2021): 713–26. https://doi.org/10.1007/s10902-021-00420-2.

Fastame, Maria Chiara, Marilena Ruiu, and Ilaria Mulas. "Mental Health and Religiosity in the Sardinian Blue Zone: Life Satisfaction and Optimism for Aging Well." *Journal of Religion and Health* 60 (April 21, 2021): 2450–62. https://doi.org/10.1007/s10943-021-01261-2.

Fastame, Maria Chiara, Paul Kenneth Hitchcott, Ilaria Mulas, Marilena Ruiu, and Maria Pietronilla Penna. "Resilience in Elders of the Sardinian Blue Zone: An Explorative Study." *Behavioral Sciences* 8, no. 3 (February 26, 2018): 30. https://doi.org/10.3390/bs8030030.

Fastame, Maria Chiara, Paul Kenneth Hitchcott, and Maria Pietronilla Penna. "The Impact of Leisure on Mental Health of Sardinian Elderly from the 'Blue Zone': Evidence for Ageing Well." *Aging Clinical and Experimental Research* 30 (May 16, 2017): 169–180. https://doi.org/10.1007/s40520-017-0768-x.

Flack, Kyle D., Kevin P. Davy, Matthew W. Hulver, Richard A. Winett, Madlyn I. Frisard, and Brenda M. Davy. "Aging, Resistance Training, and Diabetes Prevention." *Journal of Aging Research* 2011 (December 15, 2010). https://doi.org/10.4061/2011/127315.

Flinchbaugh, Carol L., E. Whitney G. Moore, Young K. Chang, and Douglas R. May. "Student Well-Being Interventions: The Effects of Stress Management Techniques and Gratitude Journaling in the Management Education Classroom." *Journal of Management Education* 36, no. 2 (April 1, 2012): 191–219. https://doi.org/10.1177%2F1052562911430062.

Franke, Andreas, Hermann Harder, Anna K. Orth, Sabine Zitzmann, and Manfred V. Singer. "Postprandial Walking but Not Consumption of Alcohol Digestifs or Espresso Accelerates Gastric Emptying in Healthy Volunteers." *Journal of Gastrointestinal and Liver Diseases* 17, no. 1 (March 2008): 27–31. https://pubmed.ncbi.nlm.nih.gov/18392240/.

Friedman, Jacob E., P. Darrell Neufer, and G. Lynis Dohm. "Regulation of Glycogen Resynthesis Following Exercise. Dietary Considerations." *Sports Medicine* 11, no. 4 (April 2011): 232–43. https://doi.org/10.2165/00007256-199111040-00003.

Going, Scott B. and Monica Laudermilk. "Osteoporosis and Strength Training." *American Journal of Lifestyle Medicine* 3, no. 4 (July 1, 2009): 310–19. https://doi.org/10.1177%2F1559827609334979.

Greiwe, Jeffrey S., Bo Cheng, Deborah C. Rubin, Kevin E. Yarasheski, and Clay F. Semenkovich. "Resistance Exercise Decreases Skeletal Muscle Tumor Necrosis Factor Alpha in Frail Elderly Humans." *The FASEB Journal* 15, no. 2 (February 2011): 475–82. https://doi.org/10.1096/fj.00-0274com.

Gutin, B. and M. J. Kasper. "Can Vigorous Exercise Play a Role in Osteoporosis Prevention? A Review." *Osteoporosis International* 2, no. 2 (March 1992): 55–69. https://doi.org/10.1007/bf01623838.

Hackney, Kyle J., Hermann-J Engles, and Randall J. Gretabeck. "Resting Energy Expenditure and Delayed-Onset Muscle Soreness After Full-Body Resistance Training with an Eccentric Concentration." *The Journal of Strength and Conditioning Research* 22, no. 5 (September 2008): 1602–9. https://doi.org/10.1519/jsc.0b013e31818222c5.

Haff, Gregory G., Alexander J. Koch, Jeffrey A. Potteiger, Karen E. Kuphal, Lawrence M. Magee, Samuel B. Green, and John J. Jakicic. "Carbohydrate Supplementation Attenuates Muscle Glycogen Loss During Acute Bouts of Resistance Exercise." *International Journal of Sport Nutrition and Exercise Metabolism* 10, no. 3 (September 2000): 326–39. https://doi.org/10.1123/ijsnem.10.3.326.

Haff, Gregory G., Mark J. Lehmkuhl, Lora B. McCoy, and Michael H. Stone. "Carbohydrate Supplementation and Resistance Training." *The Journal of Strength and Conditioning Research* 17, no. 1 (February 2003): 187–96. https://doi.org/10.1519/1533-4287(2003)017%3C0187:csart%3E2.0.co;2.

Harris, Leanne, Sharon Hamilton, Liane B. Azevedo, Joan Olajide, Caroline De Brún, Gillian Waller, Vicki Whittaker, Tracey Sharp, Mike Lean, Catherine Hankey, and Louisa Ells. "Intermittent Fasting Interventions for Treatment of Overweight and Obesity in Adults: A Systematic Review and Meta-Analysis." *JBI Database of Systematic Reviews and Implementation Reports* 16, no. 2 (February 2018): 507–47. https://doi.org/10.11124/jbisrir-2016-003248.

Harvie, Michelle, Claire Wright, Mary Pegington, Debbie McMullan, Ellen Mitchell, Bronwen Martin, Roy G. Cutler, Gareth Evans, Sigrid Whiteside, Stuart Maudsley, Simonetta Camandola, Rui Wang, Olga D. Carlson, Josephine M. Egan, Mark P. Mattson, and Anthony Howell. "The Effect of Intermittent Energy and Carbohydrate Restriction v. Daily Energy Restriction on Weight Loss and Metabolic Disease Risk Markers in Overweight Women." *British Journal of Nutrition* 110, no. 8 (October 2013): 1534–47. https://doi.org/10.1017/s0007114513000792.

Heden, Timothy, Curt Lox, Paul Rose, Steven Reid, and Erik P. Kirk. "One-Set Resistance Training Elevates Energy Expenditure for 72 H Similar to Three Sets." *European Journal of Applied Physiology* 111, no. 3 (March 2011): 477–84. https://doi.org/10.1007/s00421-010-1666-5.

Helms, Eric R., Alan A. Aragon, and Peter J. Fitschen. "Evidence-Based Recommendations for Natural Bodybuilding Contest Preparation: Nutrition and Supplementation." *Journal of the International Society of Sports and Nutrition* 11 (May 12, 2014): 20. https://doi.org/10.1186/1550-2783-11-20.

Henwood, Tim R. and Dennis R. Taaffe. "Improved Physical Performance in Older Adults Undertaking a Short-Term Programme of High-Velocity Resistance Training." *Gerontology* 51, no. 2 (March–April 2005): 108–15. https://doi.org/10.1159/000082195.

Hirotsu, Camila, Sergio Tufik, and Monica Levy Andersen. "Interactions Between Sleep, Stress, and Metabolism: From Physiological to Pathological Conditions." *Sleep Science* 8, no. 3 (November 2015): 143–52. https://doi.org/10.1016/j.slsci.2015.09.002.

Holviala, Jarkko H. S., Janne M. Sallinen, William J. Kraemer, Markku J. Alen, and Keijo K. T. Häkkinen. "Effects of Strength Training on Muscle Strength Characteristics, Functional Capabilities, and Balance in Middle-Aged and Older Women." *The Journal of Strength and Conditioning Research* 20, no. 2 (May 2006): 336–44. https://doi.org/10.1519/r-17885.1.

Hunter, Gary R., Carla J. Wetzstein, David A. Fields, Amanda Brown, and Marcas M. Bamman. "Resistance Training Increases Total Energy Expenditure and Free-Living Physical Activity in Older Adults." *Journal of Applied Physiology* 89, no. 3 (September 2000): 977–84. https://doi.org/10.1152/jappl.2000.89.3.977.

Hunter, Gary R., David R. Bryan, Carla J. Wetzstein, Paul A. Zuckerman, and Marcas M. Bamman. "Resistance Training and Intra-Abdominal Adipose Tissue in Older Men and Women." *Medicine & Science in Sports & Exercise* 34, no. 6 (June 2002): 1023–28. https://doi.org/10.1097/00005768-200206000-00019.

Hurley, Ben F., Erik D. Hanson, and Andrew K. Sheaff. "Strength Training as a Countermeasure to Aging Muscle and Chronic Disease." *Sports Medicine* 41, no. 4 (April 1, 2011): 289–306. https://doi.org/10.2165/11585920-000000000-00000.

Ibañez, Javier, Mikel Izquierdo, Iñaki Argüelles, Luis Forga, José L. Larrión, Marisol García-Unciti, Fernando Idoate, and Esteban M. Gorostiaga. "Twice-Weekly Progressive Resistance Training Decreases Abdominal Fat and Improves Insulin Sensitivity in Older Men with Type 2 Diabetes." *Diabetes Care* 28, no. 3 (March 2005): 662–67. https://doi.org/10.2337/diacare.28.3.662.

Ihalainen, Johanna K., Alistair Inglis, Tuomas Mäkinen, Robert U. Newton, Heikki Kainulainen, Heikki Kyröläinen, and Simon Walker. "Strength Training Improves Metabolic Health Markers in Older Individual Regardless of Training Frequency." *Frontiers in Physiology* 10 (February 1, 2019): 32. https://doi.org/10.3389/fphys.2019.00032.

Iwao, S., K. Mori, and Y. Sato. "Effects of Meal Frequency on Body Composition During Weight Control in Boxers." *Scandinavian Journal of Medicine & Science in Sports* 6, no. 5 (October 1996): 265–72. https://doi.org/10.1111/j.1600-0838.1996.tb00469.x.

Kalapotharakos, Vasilios I., Maria Michalopoulos, Savvas P. Tokmakidis, George Godolias, and Vasilios Gourgoulis. "Effects of a Heavy and Moderate Resistance Training on Functional Performance in Older Adults." *The Journal of Strength and Conditioning Research* 19, no. 3 (August 2005): 652–57. https://doi.org/10.1519/15284.1.

Katzmarzyk, Peter T., Timothy S. Church, Cora L. Craig, and Claude Bouchard. "Sitting Time and Mortality from All Causes, Cardiovascular Disease, and Cancer." *Medicine & Science in Sports & Exercise* 41, no. 5 (May 2009): 998–1005. https://doi.org/10.1249/mss.0b013e3181930355.

Kemmler, Wolfgang, Simon von Stengel, Jürgen Weineck, Dirk Lauber, Willi Kalender, and Klaus Engelke. "Exercise Effects on Menopausal Risk Factors of Early Postmenopausal Women: 3-Yr Erlangen Fitness Osteoporosis Prevention Study Results." *Medicine & Science in Sports & Exercise* 37, no. 2 (February 2005): 194–203. https://doi.org/10.1249/01.mss.0000152678.20239.76.

Keys, A., H. L. Taylor, F. Grande. "Basal Metabolism and Age of Adult Man." *Metabolism* 22, no. 4 (April 1973): 579–87. https://doi.org/10.1016/0026-0495(73)90071-1.

Khanijow, Vikesh, Pia Prakash, Helene A. Emsellem, Marie L. Borum, and David B. Doman. "Sleep Dysfunction and Gastrointestinal Disorders." *Gastroenterology & Hepatology* 11, no. 12 (December 2015): 817–25. https://pubmed.ncbi.nlm.nih.gov/27134599/.

Kulik, Justin R., Chad D. Touchberry, Naoki Kawamori, Peter A. Blumert, Aaron J. Crum, and G. Gregory Haff. "Supplemental Carbohydrate Ingestion Does Not Improve Performance of High-Intensity Resistance Exercise." *The Journal of Strength and Conditioning Research* 22, no. 4 (July 2008): 1101–07. https://doi.org/10.1519/jsc.0b013e31816d679b.

Lai, Chih-Chin, Yu-Kang Tu, Tyng-Guey Wang, Yi-Ting Huang, and Kuo-Liong Chien. "Effects of Resistance Training, Endurance Training and Whole-Body Vibration On Lean Body Mass, Muscle Strength and Physical Performance in Older People: A Systematic Review and Network Meta-Analysis." *Age and Ageing* 47, no. 3 (May 2018): 367–73. https://doi.org/10.1093/ageing/afy009.

Layne, Jennifer E. and Miriam E. Nelson. "The Effects of Progressive Resistance Training on Bone Density: A Review." *Medicine & Science in Sports & Exercise* 31, no. 1 (January 1999): 25–30. https://doi.org/10.1097/00005768-199901000-00006.

Legrand, Romain, Gilles Nuemi, Michel Poulain, and Patrick Manckoundia. "Description of Lifestyle, Including Social Life, Diet and Physical Activity, of People ≥90 Years Living in Ikaria, a Longevity Blue Zone." *International Journal of Environmental Research and Public Health* 18, no. 12 (June 19, 2021): 6602. https://doi.org/10.3390/ijerph18126602.

Leidy, Heather J., Cheryl L. H. Armstrong, Minghua Tang, Richard D. Mattes, and Wayne W. Campbell. "The Influence of Higher Protein Intake and Greater Eating Frequency on Appetite Control in Overweight and Obese Men." *Obesity (Silver Spring)* 18, no. 9 (September 2010): 1725–32. https://doi.org/10.1038/oby.2010.45.

Lemmer, Jeffrey T., Frederick M. Ivey, Alice S. Ryan, Greg F. Martel, Diane E. Hurlbut, J. E. Metter, Jeffre L. Fozard, James L. Fleg, and Ben F. Hurley. "Effect of Strength Training on Resting Metabolic Rate and Physical Activity: Age and Gender Comparisons." *Medicine & Science in Sports & Exercise* 33, no. 4 (April 2001): 532–41. https://doi.org/10.1097/00005768-200104000-00005.

Leproult, Rachel and Eve Van Cauter. "Effect of 1 Week of Sleep Restriction on Testosterone Levels in Young Healthy Men." *JAMA* 305, no. 21 (June 1, 2011): 2173–74. https://doi.org/10.1001/jama.2011.710.

Levine, James A., Norman L. Eberhardt, and Michael D. Jensen. "Role of Nonexercise Activity Thermogenesis in Resistance to Fat Gain in Humans." *Science* 283, no. 5399 (January 8, 1999): 212–14. https://doi.org/10.1126/science.283.5399.212.

Lopez, Michael J, and Shamim S Mohiuddin. "Biochemistry, Essential Amino Acids." National Library of Medicine, March 18, 2022. https://www.ncbi.nlm.nih.gov/books/NBK557845/.

Loucks, Anne B. and Mark Verdun. "Slow Restoration of LH Pulsatility by Refeeding in Energetically Disrupted Women." *American Journal of Physiology* 275, no. 4 (October 1998): R1218–26. https://doi.org/10.1152/ajpregu.1998.275.4.r1218.

Manson, JoAnn E., Frank B. Hu, Janet W. Rich-Edwards, Graham A. Colditz, Meir J. Stampfer, Walter C. Willett, Frank E. Speizer, and Charles H. Hennekens. "A Prospective Study of Walking as Compared With Vigorous Exercise in the Prevention of Coronary Heart Disease in Women." *The New England Journal of Medicine* 341, no. 9 (August 26, 1999): 650–58. https://doi.org/10.1056/nejm199908263410904.

Marcell, Taylor J. "Sarcopenia: Causes, Consequences, and Preventions." *The Journals of Gerontology: Series A, Biological Sciences and Medical Sciences* 58, no. 10 (October 2003): M911–16. https://doi.org/10.1093/gerona/58.10.m911.

Marston, Hannah R., Kelly Niles-Yokum, and Paula Alexandra Silva. "A Commentary on Blue Zones®: A Critical Review of Age-Friendly Environments in the 21st Century and Beyond." *International Journal of Environmental Research and Public Health* 18, no. 2 (January 19, 2021): 837. https://doi.org/10.3390/ijerph18020837.

Martin, Lily, Renate Oepen, Katharina Bauer, Alina Nottensteiner, Katja Mergheim, Harald Gruber, and Sabine C. Koch. "Creative Arts Interventions for Stress Management and Prevention—A Systematic Review." *Behavioral Sciences* 8, no. 2 (February 22, 2018): 28. https://doi.org/10.3390/bs8020028.

Meerlo, P., M. Koehl, K. van der Borght, and F. W. Turek. "Sleep Restriction Alters the Hypothalamic–Pituitary–Adrenal Response to Stress." *Journal of Neuroendocrinology* 15, no. 5 (May 2002): 397–402. https://doi.org/10.1046/j.0007-1331.2002.00790.x.

Meredith, Genevive R., Donald A. Rakow, Erin R. B. Eldermire, Cecelia G. Madsen, Steven P. Shelley, and Naomi A. Sachs. "Minimum Time Dose in Nature to Positively Impact the Mental Health of College-Aged Students, and How to Measure It: A Scoping Review." *Frontiers in Psychology* 10 (January 14, 2020): 2942. https://doi.org/10.3389/fpsyg.2019.02942.

Miller, S. L. and R. R. Wolfe. "Physical Exercise as a Modulator of Adaptation to Low and High Carbohydrate and Low and High Fat Intakes." *European Journal of Clinical Nutrition* 53 (May 28, 1999): s112–s119. https://doi.org/10.1038/sj.ejcn.1600751.

Minkel, Jared, Marisa Moreta, Julianne Muto, Oo Htaik, Christopher Jones, Mathias Basner, and David Dinges. "Sleep Deprivation Potentiates HPA Axis Stress Reactivity in Healthy Adults." *Health Psychology* 33, no. 11 (November 2014): 1430–34. https://doi.org/10.1037/a0034219.

Mullington, Janet M., Norah S. Simpson, Hans K. Meier-Ewert, and Monika Haack. "Sleep Loss and Inflammation." *Best Practice & Research Clinical Endocrinology & Metabolism* 24, no. 5 (October 2010): 775–84. https://doi.org/10.1016/j.beem.2010.08.014.

Munsters, Marjet J. and Wim H. M. Saris. "Effects of Meal Frequency on Metabolic Profiles and Substrate Partitioning in Lean Healthy Males." *PLOS One* 7, no. 6 (2012): e38632. https://doi.org/10.1371%2Fjournal.pone.0038632.

Murphy, Marie H., Alan M. Nevill, Elaine M. Murtagh, and Roger
L. Holder. "The Effect of Walking on Fitness, Fatness and Resting
Blood Pressure: A Meta-Analysis of Randomised, Controlled
Trials." *Preventive Medicine* 44, no. 5 (May 2007): 377–85. https://doi.
org/10.1016/j.ypmed.2006.12.008.

Murtagh, Elaine M., Colin A. G. Boreham, and Marie H. Murphy. "Speed
and Exercise Intensity of Recreational Walkers." *Preventive Medicine* 35,
no. 4 (October 2002): 397–400. https://doi.org/10.1006/pmed.2002.1090.

Naci, Huseyin and John P. A. Ioannidis. "Comparative Effectiveness
of Exercise and Drug Interventions on Mortality Outcomes:
Metaepidemiological Study." *BMJ* (October 1, 2013): 347. https://doi.
org/10.1136/bmj.f5577.

Nedeltcheva, Arlet V. and Frank A. J. L. Scheer. "Metabolic Effects of
Sleep Disruption, Links to Obesity and Diabetes." *Current Opinion in
Endocrinology, Diabetes, and Obesity* 21, no. 4 (August 2014): 293–98.
https://doi.org/10.1097/med.0000000000000082.

Nedeltcheva, Arlet V., Jennifer M. Kilkus, Jacqueline Imperial,
Dale A. Schoeller, and Plamen D. Penev. "Insufficient Sleep
Undermines Dietary Efforts to Reduce Adiposity." *Annals of
Internal Medicine* 153, no. 7 (October 5, 2010): 435–41. https://doi.
org/10.7326/0003-4819-153-7-201010050-00006.

Nelson, Miriam E., Maria A. Fiatarone, Christina M. Morganti, Isaiah Trice,
Robert A. Greenberg, and William J. Evans. "Effects of High-Intensity
Strength Training on Multiple Risk Factors for Osteoporotic Fracture. A
Randomized Controlled Trial." *JAMA* 272, no. 24 (December 28, 1994):
1909–14. https://doi.org/10.1001/jama.1994.03520240037038.

Nilsson, Anne C., Elin M. Ostman, Jens J. Holst, and Inger M. E. Björck.
"Including Indigestible Carbohydrates in the Evening Meal of Healthy
Subjects Improves Glucose Tolerance, Lowers Inflammatory Markers,
and Increases Satiety after a Subsequent Standardized Breakfast."
Journal of Nutrition 138, no. 4 (April 2008): 732–39. https://doi.
org/10.1093/jn/138.4.732.

O'Connor, Patrick J., Matthew P. Herring, and Amanda Caravalho. "Mental Health Benefits of Strength Training in Adults." *American Journal of Lifestyle Medicine* 4, no. 5 (May 7, 2010): 377–96. https://doi.org/10.1177%2F1559827610368771.

Olson, B. R., T. Cartledge, N. Sebring, R. Defensor, and L. Nieman. "Short-Term Fasting Affects Luteinizing Hormone Secretory Dynamics but Not Reproductive Function in Normal-Weight Sedentary Women." *The Journal of Clinical Endocrinology and Metabolism* 80, no. 4 (April 1995): 1187–93. https://doi.org/10.1210/jcem.80.4.7714088.

Ong, Kwok Leung, Bernard M. Y. Cheung, Yu Bun Man, Chu Pak Lau, and Karen S. L. Lam. "Prevalence, Awareness, Treatment, and Control of Hypertension among United States Adults 1999–2004." *Hypertension* 49, no. 1 (January 2007): 69–75. https://doi.org/10.1161/01.hyp.0000252676.46043.18.

Oustric, P., C. Gibbons, K. Beaulieu, J. Blundell, and G. Finlayson. "Changes in Food Reward During Weight Management Interventions—A Systematic Review." *Obesity Reviews* 19, no. 12 (December 2018): 1642–58. https://doi.org/10.1111/obr.12754.

Palagini, Laura, Celyne H. Bastien, Donatella Marazziti, Jason G. Ellis, and Dieter Riemann. "The Key Role of Insomnia and Sleep Loss in the Dysregulation of Multiple Systems Involved in Mood Disorders: A Proposed Model." *Journal of Sleep Research* 28, no. 6 (December 2019): e12841. https://doi.org/10.1111/jsr.12841.

Pennings, Bart, Bart B. L. Groen, Jan-Willem van Dijk, Anneke de Lange, Alexandra Kiskini, Marjan Kuklinski, Joan M. G. Senden, and Luc J. C. van Loon. "Minced Beef Is More Rapidly Digested and Absorbed than Beef Steak, Resulting in Greater Postprandial Protein Retention in Older Men." *The American Journal of Clinical Nutrition* 98, no. 1 (July 2013): 121–28. https://doi.org/10.3945/ajcn.112.051201.

Peos, Jackson J., Eric R. Helms, Paul A. Fournier, James Krieger, and Amanda Sainsbury. "A 1-Week Diet Break Improves Muscle Endurance During an Intermittent Dieting Regime in Adult Athletes: A Pre-Specified Secondary Analysis of the ICECAP Trial." *PLOS One* 16, no. 1 (February 25, 2021): e0247292. https://doi.org/10.1371/journal.pone.0247292.

Phillips, Stuart M. "Resistance Exercise: Good for More than Just Grandma and Grandpa's Muscles." *Applied Physiology, Nutrition, and Metabolism* 32, no. 6 (December 2007): 1198–205. https://doi.org/10.1139/h07-129.

Phillips, Stuart M. and Richard A. Winett. "Uncomplicated Resistance Training and Health-Related Outcomes: Evidence for a Public Health Mandate." *Current Sports Medicine Reports* 9, no. 4 (July–August 2010): 208–13. https://doi.org/10.1249/jsr.0b013e3181e7da73.

Poutanen, Kaisa S., Pierre Dussort, Alfrun Erkner, Susana Fiszman, Kavita Karnik, Mette Kristensen, Cyril F. M. Marsaux, Sophie Miquel-Kergoat, Saara P. Pentikäinen, Peter Putz, Joanne L. Slavin, Robert E. Steinert, and David J. Mela. "A Review of the Characteristics of Dietary Fibers Relevant to Appetite and Energy Intake Outcomes in Human Intervention Trials." *The American Journal of Clinical Nutrition* 106, no. 3 (September 2017): 747–54. https://doi.org/10.3945/ajcn.117.157172.

Pratley, R., B. Nicklas, M. Rubin, J. Miller, A. Smith, M. Smith, B. Hurley, and A. Goldberg. "Strength Training Increases Resting Metabolic Rate and Norepinephrine Levels in Healthy 50- to 65-Yr-Old Men." *Journal of Applied Physiology* 76, no. 1 (January 1994): 133–37. https://doi.org/10.1152/jappl.1994.76.1.133.

Robbins, Rebecca, Azizi Seixas, Lillian Walton Masters, Nicholas Chanko, Fatoumata Diaby, Dorice Vieira, and Girardin Jean-Louis. "Sleep Tracking: A Systematic Review of the Research Using Commercially Available Technology." *Current Sleep Medicine Reports* 5 (July 22, 2019): 156–63. https://doi.org/10.1007/s40675-019-00150-1.

Rosenbaum, Michael, Jules Hirsch, Dympna A. Gallagher, and Rudolph L. Leibel. "Long-Term Persistence of Adaptive Thermogenesis in Subjects Who Have Maintained a Reduced Body Weight." *The American Journal of Clinical Nutrition* 88, no. 4 (October 2008): 906–12. https://doi.org/10.1093/ajcn/88.4.906.

Roy, B. D. and M. A. Tarnopolsky. "Influence of Differing Macronutrient Intakes on Muscle Glycogen Resynthesis After Resistance Exercise." *Journal of Applied Physiology* 84, no. 3 (March 1998): 890–96. https://doi.org/10.1152/jappl.1998.84.3.890.

Salfi, Federico, Marco Lauriola, Daniela Tempesta, Pierpaolo Calanna, Valentina Socci, Luigi De Gennaro, and Michele Ferrara. "Effects of Total and Partial Sleep Deprivation on Reflection Impulsivity and Risk-Taking in Deliberative Decision-Making." *Nature of Science and Sleep* 12 (May 27, 2020): 309–24. https://doi.org/10.2147/nss.s250586.

Schlicht, Jeffrey, David N. Camaione, and Steven V. Owen. "Effect of Intense Strength Training on Standing Balance, Walking Speed, and Sit-to-Stand Performance in Older Adults." *The Journals of Gerontology: Series A, Biological Sciences and Medical Sciences* 56, no. 5 (May 2001): M281–86. https://doi.org/10.1093/gerona/56.5.m281.

Schmitz Kathryn H., Peter J. Hannan, Steven D. Stovitz, Cathy J. Bryan, Meghan Warren, and Michael D. Jensen. "Strength Training and Adiposity in Premenopausal Women: Strong, Healthy, and Empowered Study." *The American Journal of Clinical Nutrition* 86, no. 3 (September 2007): 566–72. https://doi.org/10.1093/ajcn/86.3.566.

Schoenfeld, Brad Jon, Alan Albert Aragon, and James W. Krieger. "The Effect of Protein Timing on Muscle Strength and Hypertrophy: A Meta-Analysis." *Journal of the International Society of Sports Nutrition* 10 (December 3, 2013). https://doi.org/10.1186/1550-2783-10-53.

Schoenfeld, Brad Jon, Alan Albert Aragon, and James W. Krieger. "Effects of Meal Frequency on Weight Loss and Body Composition: A Meta-Analysis." *Nutrition Reviews* 73, no. 2 (February 2015): 69–82. https://doi.org/10.1093/nutrit/nuu017.

Seimon, Radhika V., Jessica A. Roekenes, Jessica Zibellini, Benjamin Zhu, Alice A. Gibson, Andrew P. Hills, Rachel E. Wood, Neil A. King, Nuala M. Byrne, and Amanda Sainsbury. "Do Intermittent Diets Provide Physiological Benefits Over Continuous Diets for Weight Loss? A Systematic Review of Clinical Trials." *Molecular and Cellular Endocrinology* 418 part 2 (December 15, 2015): 153–72. https://doi.org/10.1016/j.mce.2015.09.014.

Snyder, Ann C., Karl Moorhead, Jacqueline Luedtke, and Mark Small. "Carbohydrate Consumption Prior to Repeated Bouts of High-Intensity Exercise." *European Journal of Applied Physiology and Occupational Physiology* 66, no. 2 (1993): 141–45. https://doi.org/10.1007/bf01427055.

Spiegel, Karine, Esra Tasali, Plamen Penev, and Eve Van Cauter. "Brief Communication: Sleep Curtailment in Healthy Young Men Is Associated with Decreased Leptin Levels, Elevated Ghrelin Levels, and Increased Hunger and Appetite." *Annals of Internal Medicine* 141, no. 11 (December 7, 2004): 846–50. https://doi.org/10.7326/0003-4819-141-11-200412070-00008.

Stote, Kim S., David J. Baer, Karen Spears, David R. Paul, G. Keith Harris, William V. Rumpler, Pilar Strycula, Samer S. Najjar, Luigi Ferrucci, Donald K. Ingram, Dan L. Longo, and Mark P. Mattson. "A Controlled Trial of Reduced Meal Frequency Without Caloric Restriction in Healthy, Normal-Weight, Middle-Aged Adults." *The American Journal of Clinical Nutrition* 85, no. 4 (April 2007): 981–88. https://doi.org/10.1093/ajcn/85.4.981.

Strasser, Barbara, Uwe Siebert, and Wolfgang Schobersberger. "Resistance Training in the Treatment of the Metabolic Syndrome: A Systematic Review and Meta-Analysis of the Effect of Resistance Training on Metabolic Clustering in Patients with Abnormal Glucose Metabolism." *Sports Medicine* 40, no. 5 (May 1, 2010): 397–415. https://doi.org/10.2165/11531380-000000000-00000.

Strasser, Barbara and Wolfgang Schobersberger, "Evidence for Resistance Training as a Treatment Therapy in Obesity." *Journal of Obesity* 2011 (August 10, 2010). https://doi.org/10.1155/2011/482564.

Taylor, M. A. and J. S. Garrow. "Compared with Nibbling, Neither Gorging nor a Morning Fast Affect Short-Term Energy Balance in Obese Patients in a Chamber Calorimeter." *International Journal of Obesity and Related Metabolic Disorders* 25, no. 4 (April 2001): 519–28. https://doi.org/10.1038/sj.ijo.0801572.

Treuth, M. S., A. S. Ryan, R. E. Pratley, M. A. Rubin, J. P. Miller, B. J. Nicklas, J. Sorkin, S. M. Harman, A. P. Goldberg, and B. F. Hurley. "Effects of Strength Training on Total and Regional Body Composition in Older Men." *Journal of Applied Physiology* 77, no. 2 (August 1994): 614–20. https://doi.org/10.1152/jappl.1994.77.2.614.

Treuth, M. S., G. R. Hunter, T. Kekes-Szabo, R. L. Weinsier, M. I, Goran, and L. Berland. "Reduction in Intra-Abdominal Adipose Tissue after Strength Training in Older Women." *Journal of Applied Physiology* 78, no. 4 (April 1995): 1425–31. https://doi.org/10.1152/jappl.1995.78.4.1425.

Tsintzas, K., C. Williams, D. Constantin-Teodosiu, E. Hultman, L. Boobis, and P. Greenhaff. "Carbohydrate Ingestion Prior to Exercise Augments the Exercise-Induced Activation of the Pyruvate Dehydrogenase Complex in Human Skeletal Muscle." *Experimental Physiology* 85, no. 5 (September 2000): 581–86. http://dx.doi.org/10.1111/j.1469-445X.2000.02043.x.

Van Etten, Ludo M. L. A., Klaas R. Westerterp, Frans T. Verstappen, Bart J. Boon, and Wim H. Saris. "Effect of an 18-Wk Weight-Training Program on Energy Expenditure and Physical Activity." *Journal of Applied Physiology* 82, no. 1 (January 1997): 298–304. https://doi.org/10.1152/jappl.1997.82.1.298.

Varady, K. A. "Intermittent Versus Daily Calorie Restriction: Which Diet Regimen Is More Effective for Weight Loss?" *Obesity Reviews* 12, no. 7 (March 2011): e593–601. http://dx.doi.org/10.1111/j.1467-789X.2011.00873.x.

Varvogli, L. and C. Darviri. "Stress Management Techniques: Evidence-Based Procedures That Reduce Stress and Promote Health." *Health Science Journal* 5, no. 2 (April 2011): 74–89. https://www.semanticscholar.org/paper/Stress-management-techniques%3A-evidence-based-that-Varvogli-Darviri/69e1ce17641b1d6b3b8c1cb3079ad741f3c9cb82.

Warren, Meghan, Moira A. Petit, Peter J. Hannan, and Kathryn H. Schmitz. "Strength Training Effects on Bone Mineral Content and Density in Premenopausal Women." *Medicine & Science in Sports & Exercise* 40, no. 7 (July 2008): 1282–88. https://doi.org/10.1249/mss.0b013e31816bce8a.

Westcott, Wayne L. "Strength Training for Frail Older Adults." *The Journal on Active Aging* (July–August 2009): 52.

Westcott, Wayne L., Richard A. Winett, James J. Annesi, Janet R. Wojcik, Eileen S. Anderson, and Patrick J. Madden. "Prescribing Physical Activity: Applying the ACSM Protocols for Exercise Type, Intensity, and Duration Across 3 Training Frequencies." *The Physician and Sportsmedicine* 37, no. 2 (June 2009): 51–58. https://doi.org/10.3810/psm.2009.06.1709.

Westerterp-Plantenga, Margriet S. "Protein Intake and Energy Balance." *Regulatory Peptides* 149, no. 1–3 (August 7, 2008): 67–69. https://doi.org/10.1016/j.regpep.2007.08.026.

Westerterp-Plantenga, Margriet S. "The Significance of Protein in Food Intake and Body Weight Regulation." *Current Opinion in Clinical Nutrition and Metabolic Care* 6, no. 6 (November 2003): 635–38. https://doi.org/10.1097/00075197-200311000-00005.

Wing, Rena R. and Robert W. Jeffery. "Prescribed 'Breaks' as a Means to Disrupt Weight Control Efforts." *Obesity Research & Clinical Practice* 11, no. 2 (February 2003): 287–91. https://doi.org/10.1038/oby.2003.43.

Wolfe, Robert R. "The Underappreciated Role of Muscle in Health and Disease." *The American Journal of Clinical Nutrition* 84, no. 3 (September 2006): 475–82. https://doi.org/10.1093/ajcn/84.3.475.

Yau, Y. H. C. and M. N. Potenza. "Stress and Eating Behaviors." *Minerva Endocrinology* 38, no. 3 (September 2013): 255–67. https://pubmed.ncbi.nlm.nih.gov/24126546/.

NOTES

1   Erin Fothergill et al., "Persistent Metabolic Adaptation 6 Years after 'The Biggest Loser' Competition,"
Obesity 24, no. 8 (August 2016): 1612–19, https://doi.org/10.1002/oby.21538.

2   Kevin D. Hall and Scott Kahan, "Maintenance of Lost Weight and Long-Term Management of Obesity,"
Medical Clinics of North America 102, no. 1 (January 2018), https://doi.org/10.1016/j.mcna.2017.08.012.

3   "About the National Health and Nutrition Examination Survey," National Health and Nutrition
Examination Survey, Centers for Disease Control and Prevention, last reviewed September 15, 2017,
https://www.cdc.gov/nchs/nhanes/about_nhanes.htm.

4   Lulu Hunt Peters, *Diet and Health: With Key to the Calories* (Chicago: Reilly & Britton, 1918).

5   Narinder Kaur, Vishal Chugh, and Anil K. Gupta, "Essential Fatty Acids as Functional Components of
Foods—A Review," *Journal of Food Science and Technology* 51, no. 10 (October 2014): 2289–303, https://
doi.org/10.1007/s13197-012-0677-0.

6   Kaur, Chugh, and Gupta, "Essential Fatty Acids."

7   Abeba Haile Mariamenatu and Emebet Mohammed Abdu, "Overconsumption of Omega-6
Polyunsaturated Fatty Acids (PUFAs) versus Deficiency of Omega-3 PUFAs in Modern-Day Diets: The
Disturbing Factor for Their 'Balanced Antagonistic Metabolic Functions' in the Human Body," *Journal of
Lipid Research* (March 2021), https://doi.org/10.1155/2021/8848161.

8   Joseph Whittaker and Kexin Wu, "Low-Fat Diets and Testosterone in Men: Systematic Review and Meta-
Analysis of Intervention Studies," *The Journal of Steroid Biochemistry and Molecular Biology* 210 (June
2021), https://doi.org/10.1016/j.jsbmb.2021.105878; D. M. Ingram et al., "Effect of Low-Fat Diet on Female
Sex Hormone Levels," *Journal of the National Cancer Institute* 79, no. 6 (December 1987): 1225–29, https://
pubmed.ncbi.nlm.nih.gov/3480374/.

9 Lopez, Michael J, and Shamim S Mohiuddin. "Biochemistry, Essential Amino Acids." National Library of Medicine, March 18, 2022. https://www.ncbi.nlm.nih.gov/books/NBK557845/.

10 Yongqing Hou and Guoyao Wu, "Nutritionally Essential Amino Acids," *Advances in Nutrition* 9, no. 6 (September 15, 2018): 849–51, https://doi.org/10.1093/advances/nmy054.

11 Jose Antonio et al., "The Effects of Consuming a High Protein Diet (4.4 g/kg/d) on Body Composition in Resistance-Trained Individuals," *Journal of the International Society of Sports Nutrition* 11 (May 12, 2014), https://doi.org/10.1186/1550-2783-11-19.

12 George A. Bray et al., "Effect of Dietary Protein Content on Weight Gain, Energy Expenditure, and Body Composition During Overeating: A Randomized Controlled Trial," *Journal of the American Medical Association* 307 (January 4, 2012): 47–55, https://doi.org/10.1001/jama.2011.1918.

13 Michaela C. Devries et al., "Changes in Kidney Function Do Not Differ Between Healthy Adults Consuming Higher- Compared with Lower- or Normal-Protein Diets: A Systematic Review and Meta-Analysis," *Journal of Nutrition* 148 (November 1, 2018): 1760–75, https://doi.org/10.1093/jn/nxy197.

14 Karen Hardy et al., "The Importance of Dietary Carbohydrate in Human Evolution," *The Quarterly Review of Biology* 90, no. 3 (September 2015): 251–68, https://doi.org/10.1086/682587.

15 David S. Ludwig, "Dietary Carbohydrates: Role of Quality and Quantity in Chronic Disease," *BMJ* 361 (June 13, 2018), https://doi.org/10.1136/bmj.k2340.

16 Herman Pontzer et al., "Hunter-Gatherer Energetics and Human Obesity," *PLOS One* 7 (July 25, 2012), https://doi.org/10.1371/journal.pone.0040503.

17 Amanda N. Szabo, "The Midwest Exercise Trial for the Prevention of Weight Regain," *Contemporary Clinical Trials* 36, no. 2 (November 2013): 470–78, https://doi.org/10.1016/j.cct.2013.08.011; Stephen D. Herrmann, "Energy Intake, Nonexercise Physical Activity, and Weight Loss in Responders and Nonresponders: The Midwest Exercise Trial 2," *Obesity* 23, no. 8 (August 2015): 1539–49, https://doi.org/10.1002/oby.21073.

18 James Clear, Atomic Habits: An Easy & Proven Way to Build Good Habits & Break Bad Ones (New York City: Avery, 2018).

19 Alia J. Crum and Ellen J. Langer, "Mind-Set Matters: Exercise and the Placebo Effect," *Psychological Science* 18, no. 2 (February 1, 2007), https://doi.org/10.1111/j.1467-9280.2007.01867.x.

20 J. Bruce Moseley et al., "A Controlled Trial of Arthroscopic Surgery for Osteoarthritis of the Knee," *The New England Journal of Medicine* 347 (July 11, 2002), https://doi.org/10.1056/nejmoa013259.

21 Paddy C. Dempsey, "Benefits for Type 2 Diabetes of Interrupting Prolonged Sitting with Brief Bouts of Light Walking or Simple Resistance Activities," *Diabetes Care* 39, no. 6 (June 2016): 964–72, https://doi.org/10.2337/dc15-2336.

22   Hye-Ryun Hong et al., "Effect of Walking Exercise on Abdominal Fat, Insulin Resistance and Serum Cytokines in Obese Women," *Journal of Exercise Nutrition and Biochemistry* 18, no. 3 (September 2014): 277–85, https://doi.org/10.5717/jenb.2014.18.3.277.

23   Sarah Hanson and Andy Jones, "Is There Evidence That Walking Groups Have Health Benefits? A Systematic Review and Meta-Analysis," *British Journal of Sports Medicine* 49, no. 11 (June 2015): 710–15, https://doi.org/10.1136/bjsports-2014-094157.

24   *Kung Fu Panda*, directed by Mark Osborne and John Stevenson (Glendale, CA: DreamWorks Animation and Dragon Warrior Media, 2008).

25   Martina de Witte et al., "Effects of Music Interventions on Stress-Related Outcomes: A Systematic Review and Two Meta-Analyses," *Health Psychology Review* 14, no. 2 (June 2020): 294–324, https://doi.org/10.108 0/17437199.2019.1627897.

26   Math Janssen et al., "Effects of Mindfulness-Based Stress Reduction on Employees' Mental Health: A Systematic Review," *PLOS One* 13, no. 1 (January 24, 2018), https://doi.org/10.1371/journal.pone.0191332.

27   Ewert, Alan, and Yun Chang. "Levels of Nature and Stress Response." National Library of Medicine, May 17, 2018. https://www.ncbi.nlm.nih.gov/pmc/articles/PMC5981243/.

28   Paul Kenneth Hitchcott et al., "Psychological Well-Being in Italian Families: An Exploratory Approach to the Study of Mental Health Across the Adult Life Span in the Blue Zone," *Europe's Journal of Psychology* 13, no. 3 (August 2017): 441–54, https://doi.org/10.5964/ejop.v13i3.1416.

29   Dan Buettner and Sam Skemp, "Blue Zones: Lessons from the World's Longest Lived," *American Journal of Lifestyle Medicine* 10, no. 5 (March 21, 2016), https://doi.org/10.1177%2F1559827616637066; Michel Poulain, Anne Herm, and Gianni Pes, "The Blue Zones: Areas of Exceptional Longevity Around the World," *Vienna Yearbook of Population Research* 11 (2013): 87–108, http://www.jstor.org/stable/43050798.

30   Darlene A. Kertes et al., "Effect of Pet Dogs on Children's Perceived Stress and Cortisol Stress Response," *Social Development* 26, no. 2 (May 2017): 382–401, https://doi.org/10.1111/sode.12203.

31   Stijn Soenen and Margriet S. Westerterp-Plantenga, "Proteins and Satiety: Implications for Weight Management," *Current Opinion in Clinical Nutrition and Metabolic Care* 11, no. 6 (November 2008): 747–51, https://doi.org/10.1097/mco.0b013e328311a8c4.

32   Dominik H. Pesta and Varman T. Samuel, "A High-Protein Diet for Reducing Body Fat: Mechanisms and Possible Caveats," *Nutrition & Metabolism* 11 (November 19, 2014), https://doi.org/10.1186/1743-7075-11-53; Jaecheol Moon and Gwanpyo Koh, "Clinical Evidence and Mechanisms of High-Protein Diet-Induced Weight Loss," *Journal of Obesity and Metabolic Syndrome* 29, no. 3 (September 30, 2020): 166–73, https://doi.org/10.7570/jomes20028; Shawn Stevenson, *Eat Smarter: Use the Power of Food to Reboot Your Metabolism, Upgrade Your Brain, and Transform Your Life* (Boston: Little, Brown and Company, 2020).

33   Heather J. Leidy et al., "Neural Responses to Visual Food Stimuli After a Normal vs. Higher Protein Breakfast in Breakfast-Skipping Teens: A Pilot fMRI Study," *Obesity (Silver Spring)* 19, no. 10 (October 2011): 2019–25, https://doi.org/10.1038/oby.2011.108.

34   Douglas Paddon-Jones et al., "Protein, Weight Management, and Satiety," *The American Journal of Clinical Nutrition* 87, no. 5 (May 2008): 1558S–61S, https://doi.org/10.1093/ajcn/87.5.1558s.

35   Thomas L. Halton and Frank B. Hu, "The Effects of High Protein Diets on Thermogenesis, Satiety and Weight Loss: A Critical Review," *Journal of the American College of Nutrition* 23, no. 5 (October 2004): 373–85, https://doi.org/10.1080/07315724.2004.10719381.

36   M. Veldhorst et al., "Protein-Induced Satiety: Effects and Mechanisms of Different Proteins," *Physiology & Behavior* 94, no. 2 (May 23, 2008): 300–307, https://doi.org/10.1016/j.physbeh.2008.01.003.

37   Heather J. Leidy et al., "Higher Protein Intake Preserves Lean Mass and Satiety with Weight Loss in Pre-Obese and Obese Women," *Obesity (Silver Spring)* 15, no. 2 (February 2007): 421–29, https://doi.org/10.1038/oby.2007.531; A. R. Skov et al., "Randomized Trial on Protein vs. Carbohydrate in ad Libitum Fat Reduced Diet for the Treatment of Obesity," *International Journal of Obesity and Related Metabolic Disorders* 23, no. 5 (May 1999): 528–36, https://doi.org/10.1038/sj.ijo.0800867; David S. Weigle, "A High-Protein Diet Induces Sustained Reductions in Appetite, ad Libitum Caloric Intake, and Body Weight Despite Compensatory Changes in Diurnal Plasma Leptin and Ghrelin Concentrations," *The American Journal of Clinical Nutrition* 82, no. 1 (July 2005): 41–48, https://doi.org/10.1093/ajcn.82.1.41.

38   M. S. Westerterp-Plantenga et al., "High Protein Intake Sustains Weight Maintenance After Body Weight Loss in Humans," *International Journal of Obesity and Related Metabolic Disorders* 28, no. 1 (January 2004): 57–64, https://doi.org/10.1038/sj.ijo.0802461.

39   Nerys M. Astbury et al., "Dose-Response Effect of a Whey Protein Preload on Within-Day Energy Intake in Lean Subjects," *British Journal of Nutrition* 104, no. 12 (December 2010): 1858–67, https://doi.org/10.1017/s000711451000293x; Lucy Chambers, Keri McCrickerd, and Martin R. Yeomans, "Optimising Foods for Satiety," *Food Science and Technology* 41, no. 2 (February 2015): 149–60, https://doi.org/10.1016/j.tifs.2014.10.007.

40   R. J. Stubbs et al., "Breakfasts High in Protein, Fat or Carbohydrate: Effect on Within-Day Appetite and Energy Balance," *European Journal of Clinical Nutrition* 50, no. 7 (July 1996): 409–17, https://pubmed.ncbi.nlm.nih.gov/8862476/.

41   Stefan M. Pasiakos, Harris R. Lieberman, and Victor L. Fulgoni, III, "Higher-Protein Diets Are Associated with Higher HDL Cholesterol and Lower BMI and Waist Circumference in US Adults," *The Journal of Nutrition* 145, no. 3 (March 2015): 605–14, https://doi.org/10.3945/jn.114.205203.

42   J. L. Krok-Schoen et al., "Low Dietary Protein Intakes and Associated Dietary Patterns and Functional Limitations in an Aging Population: A NHANES Analysis," *The Journal of Nutrition, Health & Aging* 23 (February 19, 2019): 338–47, https://doi.org/10.1007/s12603-019-1174-1.

43   James M. Lattimer and Mark D. Haub, "Effects of Dietary Fiber and Its Components on Metabolic Health," *Nutrients* 2, no. 12 (December 2010): 1266–89, https://doi.org/10.3390/nu2121266.

44   Athanasios Papathanasopoulos and Michael Camilleri, "Dietary Fiber Supplements: Effects in Obesity and Metabolic Syndrome and Relationship to Gastrointestinal Functions," *Gastroenterology* 138, no. 1 (January 2010): 65–72, https://doi.org/10.1053/j.gastro.2009.11.045.

45 Ygor Parladore Silva, Andressa Bernardi, and Rudimar Luiz Frozza, "The Role of Short-Chain Fatty Acids from Gut Microbiota in Gut-Brain Communication," *Frontiers in Endocrinology* 11 (January 31, 2020): 25, https://doi.org/10.3389/fendo.2020.00025.

46 Alessia Pascale et al., "Microbiota and Metabolic Diseases," *Endocrine* 61 (May 2, 2018): 357–71, https://doi.org/10.1007/s12020-018-1605-5.

47 Ji Na Jeong, "Effect of Pre-meal Water Consumption on Energy Intake and Satiety in Non-obese Young Adults," *Clinical Nutrition Research* 7, no. 4 (October 31, 2018): 291–96, https://doi.org/10.7762/cnr.2018.7.4.291.

48 Robert A. Corney, Caroline Sunderland, and Lewis J. James, "Immediate Pre-Meal Water Ingestion Decreases Voluntary Food Intake in Lean Young Males," *European Journal of Nutrition* 55 (April 18, 2015): 815–19, https://doi.org/10.1007/s00394-015-0903-4.

49 Melissa C. Daniels and Barry M. Popkin, "Impact of Water Intake on Energy Intake and Weight Status: A Systematic Review," *Nutrition Reviews* 68, no. 9 (September 2010): 505–21, https://doi.org/10.1111/j.1753-4887.2010.00311.x.

50 Katherine Hawton et al., "Slow Down: Behavioural and Physiological Effects of Reducing Eating Rate," *Nutrients* 11, no. 1 (December 27, 2018): 50, https://doi.org/10.3390/nu11010050.

51 Eric Robinson et al., "Eating Attentively: A Systematic Review and Meta-Analysis of the Effect of Food Intake Memory and Awareness on Eating," *The American Journal of Clinical Nutrition* 97, no. 4 (April 2013): 728–42, https://doi.org/10.3945/ajcn.112.045245.

52 Eric T. Trexler, Abbie E. Smith-Ryan, and Layne E. Norton, "Metabolic Adaptation to Weight Loss: Implications for the Athlete," *Journal of the International Society of Sports Nutrition* 11, no. 1 (February 27, 2014): 7, https://doi.org/10.1186/1550-2783-11-7.

53 G. Boden et al., "Effect of Fasting on Serum Leptin in Normal Human Subjects," *The Journal of Clinical Endocrinology & Metabolism* 81, no. 9 (September 1, 1996): 3419–23, https://doi.org/10.1210/jcem.81.9.8784108; Jean L. Chan et al., "The Role of Falling Leptin Levels in the Neuroendocrine and Metabolic Adaptation to Short-Term Starvation in Healthy Men," *Journal of Clinical Investigation* 111, no. 9 (May 1, 2003): 1409–21, https://doi.org/10.1172/JCI17490.

54 Brian Kim, "Thyroid Hormone as a Determinant of Energy Expenditure and the Basal Metabolic Rate," *Thyroid* 18, no. 2 (February 2008): 141–44, https://doi.org/10.1089/thy.2007.0266.

55 Olav E. Rooyackers and K. Sreekumaran Nair, "Hormonal Regulation of Human Muscle Protein Metabolism," *Annual Review of Nutrition* 17 (July 1997): 457–85, https://doi.org/10.1146/annurev.nutr.17.1.457.

56 Rooyackers and Nair, "Hormonal Regulation."

57 Ralph E. Smith and Emmett V. Schmidt, "Induction of Anemia by Avian Leukosis Viruses of Five Subgroups," *Virology* 117, no. 2 (March 1982): 516–18, https://doi.org/10.1016/0042-6822(82)90492-5.

58   Hiroyuki Ariyasu et al., "Stomach Is a Major Source of Circulating Ghrelin, and Feeding State Determines Plasma Ghrelin-Like Immunoreactivity Levels in Humans," *The Journal of Endocrinology & Metabolism* 86, no. 10 (October 1, 2001): 4753–58, https://doi.org/10.1210/jcem.86.10.7885.

59   Chiara De Maddalena et al., "Impact of Testosterone on Body Fat Composition," *Journal of Cellular Physiology* 227, no. 12 (December 2012): 3744–48, https://doi.org/10.1002/jcp.24096.

60   De Maddalena, "Impact of Testosterone."

61   K. E. Zakrzewska et al., "Glucocorticoids as Counterregulatory Hormones of Leptin: Toward an Understanding of Leptin Resistance," *Diabetes* 46, no. 4 (1997): 717–19, https://doi.org/10.2337/diab.46.4.717.

62   Trexler, "Metabolic Adaptation to Weight Loss," studies 1, 2, 19, 28, 29, 30, and 31.

63   Trexler, "Metabolic Adaptation to Weight Loss," studies 32 and 33.

64   Trexler, "Metabolic Adaptation to Weight Loss."

65   Trexler, "Metabolic Adaptation to Weight Loss."

66   A. Sainsbury et al., "Rationale for Novel Intermittent Dieting Strategies to Attenuate Adaptive Responses to Energy Restriction," *Obesity Reviews* 19, no. S1 (December 3, 2018): 47–60, https://doi.org/10.1111/obr.12787.

67   Bill I. Campbell et al., "Intermittent Energy Restriction Attenuates the Loss of Fat Free Mass in Resistance Trained Individuals. A Randomized Controlled Trial," *Journal of Functional Morphology and Kinesiology* 5, no. 1 (March 8, 2020): 19, https://doi.org/10.3390/jfmk5010019; Jackson James Peos et al., "Intermittent Dieting: Theoretical Considerations for the Athlete," *Sports* 7, no. 1 (January 16, 2019): 22, https://doi.org/10.3390/sports7010022.

68   Campbell, "Intermittent Energy Restriction."

69   Layne Norton and Peter Baker, *Fat Loss Forever: How to Lose Fat and Keep it Off* (Self-published, BioLayne, 2019).

70   Mario Servio et al., "Efficiency of Autoregulatory Homeostatic Responses to Imposed Caloric Excess in Lean Men," *American Journal of Physiology–Endocrinology and Metabolism* 294, no. 2 (February 2008): E416–24, https://doi.org/10.1152/ajpendo.00573.2007.

71   F. Johnson, M. Pratt, and J. Wardle, "Dietary Restraint and Self-Regulation in Eating Behavior," *International Journal of Obesity* 36, no. 5 (2012): 665–74, https://doi.org/10.1038/ijo.2011.156.

72   Laurin Alexandra Conlin et al., "Flexible vs. Rigid Dieting in Resistance-Trained Individuals Seeking to Optimize Their Physiques: A Randomized Controlled Trial," *Journal of the International Society of Sports Nutrition* 18, no. 1 (April 1, 2022), https://doi.org/10.1186/s12970-021-00452-2.

73 Yue Sun et al., "Stress Triggers Flare of Inflammatory Bowel Disease in Children and Adults," *Frontiers in Pediatrics* 24, no. 7 (October 24, 2019): 432, https://doi.org/10.3389/fped.2019.00432.

74 M. Ellen Kuenzig et al., "Twenty-First Century Trends in the Global Epidemiology of Pediatric-Onset Inflammatory Bowel Disease: Systematic Review," *Gastroenterology* 162, no. 4 (April 1, 2022): 1147–59, https://doi.org/10.1053/j.gastro.2021.12.282.

75 Vanessa K. Ridaura et al., "Gut Microbiota from Twins Discordant for Obesity Modulate Metabolism in Mice," *Science* 341, no. 6150 (September 6, 2013), https://doi.org/10.1126/science.1241214.

76 Ridaura, "Gut Microbiota from Twins."

77 Wayne L. Westcott, "Resistance Training is Medicine: Effects of Strength Training on Health," *Current Sports Medicine Reports* 11, no. 4 (July–August 2012): 209–16, https://doi.org/10.1249/jsr.0b013e31825dabb8.

78 Andrew D. Williams et al., "Cardiovascular and Metabolic Effects of Community Based Resistance Training in an Older Population," *Journal of Science and Medicine in Sport* 14, no. 4 (July 2011): 331–37, https://doi.org/10.1016/j.jsams.2011.02.011.

79 Simon Melov et al., "Resistance Exercise Reverses Aging in Human Skeletal Muscle," *PLOS One* 2, no. 5 (2007): e465, https://doi.org/10.1371%2Fjournal.pone.0000465.

80 Hong, "Effect of Walking Exercise."

81 Mohammad Kazem Hosseini-Asl, Erfan Taherifard, and Mohammad Reza Mousavi, "The Effect of a Short-Term Physical Activity After Meals on Gastrointestinal Symptoms in Individuals with Functional Abdominal Bloating: A Randomized Clinical Trial," *Gastroenterology and Hepatology from Bed to Bench* 14, no. 1 (Winter 2021): 59–66, https://www.ncbi.nlm.nih.gov/pmc/articles/PMC8035544/.

Made in the USA
Las Vegas, NV
30 January 2024

85113275R00108